HANDBOOK *of*

VASCULAR

BRACHYTHERAPY

Second Edition

HANDBOOK *of*

VASCULAR

BRACHYTHERAPY

Second Edition

Edited by

Ron Waksman MD FACC
Director
Experimental Angioplasty and Vascular Brachytherapy
Cardiology Research Foundation
Washington Hospital Center
Washington DC
USA

Patrick W Serruys MD PhD FACC FESC
Professor of Interventional Cardiology
Division of Cardiology
Thoraxcenter
Academic Hospital Rotterdam-Dijkzigt
Rotterdam
The Netherlands

MARTIN DUNITZ

© Martin Dunitz Ltd 1998, 2000

First published in the United Kingdom in 1998 by
Martin Dunitz Ltd
The Livery House
7–9 Pratt Street
London NW1 0AE
Tel: +44 (0)207 482 2202
Fax: +44 (0)207 267 0159
E-mail: info@mdunitz.globalnet.co.uk
Website: http://www.dunitz.co.uk

Second Edition 2000

A CIP catalogue record for this book is available from the British Library

ISBN 1–85317–803–9

Distributed in the United States by:
Blackwell Science Inc.
Commerce Place, 350 Main Street
Malden MA 02148, USA
Tel: 1 800 215 1000

Distributed in Canada by:
Login Brothers Book Company
324 Salteaux Crescent
Winnipeg, Manitoba R3J 3T2
Canada
Tel: 1 204 224 4068

Distributed in Brazil by:
Ernesto Reichmann Distribuidora de Livros, Ltda
Rua Coronel Marques 335
03440–000 São Paulo–SP
Brazil

Composition by Scribe Design, Gillingham, Kent
Printed and bound in Spain by Grafos, S.A.

CONTENTS

LIST OF CONTRIBUTORS

Howard I Amols PhD
Columbia University
Department of Radiation Oncology
New York NY
USA

Marc G Apple MD
Parkview Radiation
Oncology Center
2500 East State Blvd
Fort Wayne IN
USA

Stephen Balter
Lenox Hill Hospital
Heart and Vascular Institute of New York,
New York, NY
USA

Raoul Bonan MD
Novoste Corporation
Norcross GA
USA

David J Brenner DSc
Center for Radiological Research
Columbia University
New York NY
USA

Maurice Buchbinder
Novoste Corporation
Norcross GA
USA

Richard V Calfee PhD
The Methodist Hospital – Houston
Cardiac Catheterization Laboratory
Houston TX
USA

Rosanna Chan
CVRT Ltd/Sorea
Yavne
Israel

Ary Chernomorsky
Vascular Therapies
Menlo Park CA
USA

Victor I Chornenky PhD
2670 Patton Road
St Paul MN
USA

Jay P Ciezki MD
Cleveland Clinic Foundation
Cleveland OH
USA

Marco A Costa MD
Thorax Center
University Hospital Dijkcigt
Emasmus University
Rotterdam
The Netherlands

Bert M Coursey PhD
National Institute of Standards and
Technology
Ionizing Radiation Division
Gaithersburg MD
USA

Richard diMonda MBA
Novoste Corporation
Norcross GA
USA

Neal Eigler MD
Cedars-Sinai Medical Center
Los Angeles CA
USA

Robert P Eno
Guidant Corporation Vascular Intervention
Houston TX
USA

David Faxon MD
Vascular Therapies
Norwalk CT
USA

David R Fischell PhD
Isostent Inc
Belmont CA
USA

Robert E Fischell DSc
Isostent Inc
Belmont CA
USA

Tim A Fischell MD FACC
Isostent Inc
Belmont CA
USA

Robert I Grove PhD
Miravant Medical Technologies
Santa Barbara CA
USA

Ross Heath
Miravant Medical Technologies
Santa Barbara CA
USA

Christoph Hehrlein
Isotent Inc
Belmont CA
USA

Richard A Hillstead PhD
Novoste Corporation
Norcross GA
USA

Shirish K Jani PhD
Scripps Clinic and Research Foundation
La Jolla CA
USA

Michael H Keelan Jr MD FACC
Division of Cardiovascular Medicine
Medical College of Wisconsin
Milwaukee WI
USA

Danny Kijel
CVRT Ltd/Sorea
Yavne
Israel

Nicholas N Kipshidze MD PhD FACC
Lenox Hill Heart and Vascular Institute,
Lenox Hill Hospital
New York, NY
USA

Efi Lavie PhD
Soreq, Nuclear Research Center
Yavne
Israel

Ian M Leitch PhD
Miravant Medical Technologies
Santa Barbara CA
USA

Sam Liprie PhD NC
Vascular Therapies
Norwalk CT
USA

Frank Litvack MD
Cedars-Sinai Medical Center
Los Angeles CA
USA

Raj Makkar MD
Cedars-Sinai Medical Center
Los Angeles CA
USA

Vincent Massullo MD
Scripps Clinic and Research Foundation
La Jolla CA
USA

Dattatreyudu Nori MD
New York Hospital Cornell Medical
Center
New York NY
USA

Suhrid Parikh PhD
New York Hospital Cornell Medical
Center
New York NY
USA

Youri G Popowski PhD
Division of Radiation Oncology
University Hospital
Geneva
Switzerland

Mark Purter
Miravant Medical Technologies
Santa Barbara CA
USA

Albert E Raizner MD
The Methodist Hospital–Houston
Cardiac Catheterization Laboratory
Houston TX
USA

Steve Rychnovsky PhD
Miravant Medical Technologies
Santa Barbara CA
USA

Manel Sabaté
Servicio de Cardiologia Intervencionista,
Hospital Clinico Universitario 'San Carlos'
Madrid
Spain

Harry Sahota MB MD
Sohata Heart Institute
Bellflower CA
USA

Eli Sayag
CVRT Ltd/Sorea
Yavne
Israel

Stephen M Seltzer MS
National Institute of Standards and
Technology
Ionizing Radiation Division
Gaithersburg MD
USA

Patrick W Serruys MD PhD
ThoraxCenter
University Hospital Dijkzigt
Erasmus University
Rotterdam
The Netherlands

Edward F Smith III
Mallinckrodt Medical
Radiance Medical Systems
Irvine CA
USA

Christopher G Soares PhD
National Institute of Standards and
Technology
Ionizing Radiation Division
Gaithersburg MD
USA

ix

Burton L Speiser MD, MS
Arizona Oncology Services
Radiation Oncology Dept
St Josephs Hospital
Phoenix, AZ
USA

Pat Stephens MS
Miravant Medical Technologies
Santa Barbara CA
USA

Gary Strathearn
Miravant Medical Technologies
Santa Barbara CA
USA

Lisa A Tam
Miravant Medical Technologies
Santa Barbara CA
USA

Paul Teirstein
Scripps Clinic and Research Foundation
La Jolla CA
USA

Brett Trauthen
Miravant Medical Technologies
Santa Barbara CA
USA

Prabhakar Tripuraneni
Scripps Clinic and Research Foundation
La Jolla CA
USA

Vitali E Verin PhD
Cardiology Center
University Hospital
Switzerland

Jeff Walker MD
Miravant Medical Technologies
Santa Barbara CA
USA

Ron Waksman MD FACC
Cardiology Research Foundation
Washington Hospital Center
Washington DC
USA

Chris Waters PhD
Miravant Medical Technologies
Santa Barbara CA
USA

Judah Weinberger MD PhD
Cardiovascular Division
Columbia Presbyterian Medical Center
New York NY
USA

James S Whiting
Cedars-Sinai Medical Center
Davies Research Building
Los Angeles CA
USA

Brian E Zimmerman PhD
National Institute of Standards and
Technology
Ionizing Radiation Division
Gaithersburg MD
USA

PREFACE

The exponential development of the field of vascular brachytherapy mandates a new edition for the *Handbook of Vascular Brachytherapy*. Two years after publishing the first edition technology, supported by positive randomized clinical trials with gamma radiation for the treatment of restenosis and encouraging data from feasibility studies utilizing beta sources in native coronaries, has progressed remarkably. Extensive research and efforts by investigators around the globe have led to better understanding of the biology, the physics and the dosimetry issues related to the field. In addition, improvements to the pioneering devices and new innovations to deliver radiation into the vessels have been introduced to the medical community. The multidisciplinary approach of cardiologists, radiation therapists, physicists, biologists, engineers and industry personel has been proven to work for this exciting technology. At the time of publication of this second edition, vascular brachytherapy is already approved for use in several European countries and close for limited marketing approval in the USA. As the technology matures, we hope to find solutions for identified complications (edge effect and late thrombosis).

The second edition of the *Handbook of Vascular Brachytherapy* brings to the medical community a practical tool to understand the fundamental terminology and components of vascular brachytherapy including radiation physics and radiation biology and an up-to-date review of the new devices designed to deliver radiation into the vessel. An update on the clinical status of the clinical trials in the USA and in Europe and some safety tips on radiation safety are also included. This second edition contains nine new chapters while the majority of the other chapters have been revised to brine you the most up-to-date practical document on vascular brachytherapy.

We would like to thank the contributors – cardiologists, radiation oncologists, medical physicists, radiobiologists, and industry representatives for their efforts to bring this book together. Alan Burgess from Martin Dunitz Publishers deserves special recognition for collecting and handling the written material most professionally to bring this second edition to press in less than five months. We thank Yasmin Khan-Chowdhury for managing the editorial process so efficiently. We sincerely hope that this book will help clinicians, researchers and engineers not only in keeping up with the new developments in this field but also to continue to look for improvements, innovative ideas and clinical implications of this technology to reach the common goal of improving patient care.

Ron Waksman
Patrick W Serruys

1. BASIC TERMS IN RADIATION, PHYSICS, ONCOLOGY, BIOLOGY AND BRACHYTHERAPY

Arizona Oncology Services, Radiation Oncology Dept, St Josephs Hospital, Phoenix, AZ, USA

Burton L Speiser

A Symbol for mass number. The sum of Z (atomic number) and N (neutron number).

Absorbed dose (D) The amount of energy of ionizing radiation delivered to matter of a defined mass and volume. The absorbed dose is the expected amount of the energy imparted to matter per unit mass at a point. The units of absorbed dose are the same as those used for kerma: the gray (Gy) or the non-SI* unit, the rad.

$$1 \text{ Gy} = 1 \text{ J kg}^{-1} = 100 \text{ rad}$$

Accelerator A device used to increase the velocity, and the energy, of atomic particles, by means of an electromagnetic field. The accelerated particles cause nuclear and other reactions in the target. Common types of accelerators are the cyclotron, synchrotron, synchrocyclotron, betatron, and van de Graaf accelerator. The most common devices are the linear accelerators used in radiation oncology.

Activation The process of inducting radioactivity. Most artificially produced radioactive substances are produced by neutron-capture reactions. This is written as

$$\frac{59}{27} \text{ co } (n,\gamma) \quad \frac{60}{27} \text{ co}$$

Activity The average number of spontaneous nuclear transitions from one energy state to a lower energy state occurring in a radionuclide, divided by that time interval. The SI† unit of activity is the becquerel (Bq); the non-SI unit is the curie (Ci).

$$1 \text{ Ci} = 3.7 \times 10^{10} \text{ disintegrations/s}$$
$$1 \text{ Ci} = 3.7 \times 10^{10} \text{ Bq}$$
$$1 \text{ Bq} = 2.7 \times 10^{-11} \text{ Ci}$$

---

*Non-SI: units used from the early twentieth century or later to the present time.
†See SI entry: SI = Systeme International.

Acute dose response A response occurring either during or within 6 months after completion of radiation treatment or acute exposure to radiation of a sufficient amount.

Alpha (α) emission Particulate radiation consisting of fast-moving helium nuclei (two rotons, two neutrons) produced by the disintegration of heavy nuclei (those with an atomic number > 52). A process of radioactive decay, where one isotope changes into another element.

Alpha (α) particle This consists of two protons and two neutrons and produces dense ionization owing to its large charge and mass, usually with an energy between 3 and 7 MeV. Owing to their heavy mass and double electronic charge, they interact strongly with surrounding atoms producing a very high density of ionizations and linear energy transfer along their track. For example, a 5-MeV α-particle creates 7000 ion pairs per mm at the start of its track (in tissue) and has a linear energy transfer of 55 keV μm^{-1}. This rapid loss of energy results in a very short range, typically < 0.1 mm. The rapid deposition of energy also results in considerable biological damage. For both these reasons, radionuclides emitting α-particles are not suitable for use in nuclear medicine.

Atom The smallest unit of an element consisting of a single nucleus surrounded by one or more orbital electrons. In a resting state, the number of electrons is sufficient to make the atom electrically neutral. Adding or removing one or more electrons turns the atom into a negative or positive ion. The atom of a given element is identified by its atomic number, which is the number of electrons about the nucleus, or conversely the number of protons in the nucleus.

Atomic mass unit (amu) This unit is used most commonly in chemistry and is equivalent to 1/16 of the mass of one neutral atom of oxygen-16; equivalent to 1.66×10^{-24} g, 931 MeV, 1.49×10^{-3} erg, or 0.999728 atomic weight units. (Weight and mass may not always be equal.)

Atomic weight The mean weight of an element's atoms, expressed in either atomic mass units (physical scale) or atomic weight units (chemical scale). All elements have several isotopes, which differ in the weights of their atoms. Therefore, the average mass of the atoms in a sample will depend on whether it is a mixture of isotopes (e.g. in their naturally occurring proportions) or a single isotope.

Attenuation The process by which a beam of radiation is reduced in intensity when passing through matter. It is the combination of absorption and scattering processes and leads to a decrease in 'strength' of the beam when projected through matter.

Attenuation coefficient Attenuation per unit length of wave travel. (Holds for all of electromagnetic radiations.)

Attenuation factor A measure of the absorptive properties of a layer of material for radiation traversing it and defined as the ratio of the incident intensity to the transmitted intensity.

Auger effect The non-radioactive transition of an atom from an excited electronic energy state to a lower state with the emission of an electron. The term refers to the x-ray region of energy states. The electron ejected in the Auger effect is known as an Auger electron.

Auger electrons Those electrons emitted from an atom owing to the filling of a vacancy in an inner electron shell.

Authorized limits Upper levels of radiation exposure of individuals. These are not levels associated with known clinical effects, rather levels with 'margins of safety'.

Beam profile The magnitude of radiation intensity as a function of position in a cross-sectional plane of a radiation beam.

Becquerel (Bq) The SI unit of radioactivity. One becquerel is equivalent to one nuclear disintegration per second. The conventional unit for radioactivity is the curie: $1\ Bq = 2.70 \times 10^{-11}\ Ci$.

Bergonie-Tribondeau law The radiosensitivity of a tissue is directly proportional to its reproductive capacity and inversely proportional to its degree of differentiation. The more primitive the cell, the greater its sensitivity within a species

Beta (β) decay The transformation of nuclei either by the spontaneous emission of electrons or positrons, or by the capture of an orbital electron from the K-shell, is known as β decay. The rate of decay is proportional to the number of nuclei present, the constant of proportionality being known as the decay constant. For all three processes the mass number of the nucleus does not change. The reaction schemes for the three processes—electron emission, positron emission, and K-capture—are:

$$Z^A \rightarrow (Z+1)^A + \beta^- \text{ electron emission}$$
$$Z^A \rightarrow (Z-1)^A + \beta^+ \text{ positron emission}$$
$$Z^A + \beta_k \rightarrow (Z-1)^A \text{ K-capture}$$

where the symbol Z^A characterizes a nucleus of atomic number Z and mass number A.

Beta emitter Any radioactive nuclide that decays by β decay with the emission of a β particle.

3

Beta-gamma emitter Beta disintegrations are sometimes accompanied by the emission of γ-rays. In such cases the emission of a β particle leads to a nucleus in an excited state, which by the emission of a γ-ray returns to its ground state.

Beta particle In 1900, Becquerel showed that β-rays could behave like the rays from a cathode tube and named these β particles, as electrons. Some of the artificially produced radioisotopes decay by emission of a positron or positive electron; the name β particle is also applied (β^- or β^+).

   β particles interact very weakly with nuclei, so they are not useful for inducing nuclear reactions. However, positive β particle, which has been slowed down sufficiently, can unite with an electron. The positron and electrons are then annihilated and the energy appears as two γ-rays, each of energy about 0.511 MeV, which is emitted in opposite directions (annihilation radiation).

Biological half-life ($T_{b1/2}$) The time required for the body to eliminate one-half of an administered dose of any substance by regular processes of elimination. This time is approximately the same for both the stable and radioactive isotopes of the same element.

Biologic effectiveness of radiation Also known as the Relative Biologic Effectiveness (RBE). This is expressed as the dose of radiation delivered to produce a specific end effect divided by the dose of a different radiation, i.e. if a radiation has an RBE of 1.5 it is 50% more effective than the radiation it is being compared to (that within the denominator).

Bohr's atomic theory The theory that atoms can exist for a duration solely in certain states characterized by definite electronic orbits, i.e. by definite energy levels of their extranuclear electrons. In these stationary states, they do not emit radiation; the jump of an electron from one orbit to another of a smaller radius is accompanied by monochromatic radiation.

Brachytherapy Brachytherapy is derived from the Greek for 'brachy' meaning short and 'therapy' meaning treatment, in which sealed sources of radioactive material are used to deliver radiation at a very short distance by placing the sources within cavities, lumens, within tissue or on the surface. The physical benefit of this mode of treatment is that very high doses of radiation can be delivered directly or almost directly to the target with a very rapid fall off of dose to the surrounding normal tissues.

Bremsstrahlung (German for braking radiation.) The electromagnetic radiation produced when an electron passes near a nucleus and is deflected from its path.

Build-up factor When radiation passes through material, the number of collisions may not be the maximum. This term refers to the addition of material to reach that level of interactions at the material's surface.

By-product material Any radioactive material yielded in or made radio-active by exposure to radiation for the purpose of producing nuclear material.

Calibration Determination of accuracy of a measuring instrument to ascertain necessary correction factors. A procedure for standardizing radiation detection instruments for various parameters, such as quantitation of the amount of radioactivity, uniformity of response, spatial resolution, etc.

Charge particles Most atomic particles carry an electrostatic charge, the exceptions being the neutron, and certain mesons. The charged particles may have either positive or negative charge, which is always one or more units of the charge of the electron ($e = 1.6 \times 10^{-19}$ C) (C = coulomb = 3×10^9 electrostatic units). The positively charged particles comprise atomic nuclei, positive electrons (positrons), and positive mesons; while the negatively charged particles are electrons, antiprotons, and negative mesons.

Chemical radiation protector A chemical agent that reduces the intensity of a particular radiation effect when added to a chemical or biological system. The agent may be added before exposure such as potassium iodide for thyroid blocking, or after exposures as with electron scavengers.

Chromatid The two halves of a chromosome that has divided longitudinally at mitosis and meiosis, and which are held together at the centromere.

Chromatin (From the Greek chroma—color.) The part of a cell nucleus which is readily stainable, composed of DNA and proteins (primarily histones), and is the primary carrier of genes.

Chromosome The thread-shaped bodies composed of chromatin in the nucleus of a cell, consisting of connected strands of DNA molecules (genes) involved in the transmission of genetic information during cell division. As the cell divides, one-half goes to the nucleus of each of the daughter cells. The number of chromosomes per cell varies greatly from organism to organism; man has 46.

Compton effect The change in wavelength for x- and γ-radiation in which the incident photon interacts with an orbital electron on the absorber atom to produce a recoil electron and a photon of energy less than the incident photon.

Compton recoil particle The accelerated electron resulting from the process of Compton scattering. Also known as Compton electron or recoil electron.

Concentrations of radioactivity Amount of radioactivity per volume unit, e.g. 1 MBq/ml (see also specific activity).

Conversion electron Orbital electron that has been excited (ionized) by internal conversion of an excited atom.

Cosmic rays High-energy particles and electromagnetic radiations, which bombard the earth from outer space. The particles hitting the outer atmosphere are mostly protons, but, as a result of collisions with atmospheric nuclei, other forms of radiation (Millikan rays, ultra x-rays) are produced with a wide range of energies and penetrating power.

Counter A detector of radiation, which gives an instantaneous, discrete, electrical signal upon passage of a particle or x- or γ-ray through it. Counters may be of various types, the most important being the pulse ionization chamber, proportional counter, Geiger–Müller (GM) counter, and scintillation counter, solid and liquid.

Curie A non-SI unit of radioactivity defined as 3.70×10^{10} disintegrations per second. One gram of radium has an activity of 1 Ci. (Abbreviated Ci, several fractions of the curie are in common usage.) The SI unit is the becquerel (one disintegration per second).

Cutie pie (Colloquial term.) Portable ionization chamber for determining relatively stable dose rates. It is an ionization chamber plus electrometer and uses the voltage-drop method.

Cyclotron Invented by EO Lawrence in 1931, the cyclotron in one or another variation is the nuclear particle accelerator of choice for the production of radioisotopes by charged particle-induced nuclear reactions. Nuclear reactors, which produce neutron-rich radioisotopes by neutron bombardment, supplanted cyclotrons in the 1950s and 1960s as the major producers of radioisotopes, but the latter are still the dominant producers of neutron-deficient radioisotopes.

Daughter product A nuclide formed by the decay of a radionuclide. A daughter product may be either radioactive or stable. Synonym for decay product.

Decay When a radioactive atom disintegrates it is said to decay; what remains is a different element. Polonium decays to form lead, ejecting an α particle in the process. In a mass of a particular radioisotope a number of atoms will disintegrate or decay every second—and this number is a characteristic of the isotope concerned.

Decay constant The fraction of the number of atoms of a radioactive nuclide, which decays in a specified time. Symbol: $\lambda = 0.693_{+1/2}$ is the half-life of a radionuclide. It may also be noted that λ is the reciprocal of the mean of average life of the radioactive nuclide.

Directly ionizing particles Charged particles having sufficient kinetic energy to produce ionization by collision.

Disintegration A spontaneous process in which the nucleus of an atom changes its form or its energy state, by emitting either particulate or electromagnetic radiation, or by electron capture.

Disintegration energy The energy that is released in the radioactive decay of a nucleus. For example, in α decay, it is the sum of the kinetic energy of the α particle and the recoil energy of the daughter nucleus, when the daughter nucleus is formed in the ground state. In nuclear reactions, the distintegration energy is more commonly termed the Q value of the reaction. The Q value may be positive or negative.

Disintegration rate The number of disintegrations per unit of time (disintegrations per second). The standard unit is the becquerel, which equals one disintegration per second.

Dose The radiation delivered to any target. This is a general term denoting the quantity of radiation or energy absorbed in a specified mass. The SI unit of absorbed dose is the gray (Gy) and the non-SI unit is the rad (1 Gy = 100 rad, 1 cGY = 1 rad). The term is also used loosely for the amount of radioactivity administered.

Dose rate The dose of radiation per unit of time (delivered or received).

Dose response curve Curve indicating percent response to specified doses.

Dose threshold The minimum absorbed dose that will produce a specified effect.

Dose volume The product of absorbed dose and the volume of the absorbing mass.

Dosimeter Instrument used to detect and measure an accumulated dosage of radiation; in common usage it is a pencil-sized ionization chamber with a built-in self-reading electrometer; used for personnel monitoring.

Effective half-life (T_e) Time required for an administered dose to be reduced to one-half, owing to both physical decay and biologic elimination of radionuclide. It is given $T_e = (T_p \times T_b)/(T_p + T_b)$, where T_e is the effective half-life, and T_p and T_b are the physical and biologic half-lives, respectively. Note: If an isotope used within the coronaries escapes into the systemic circulation, there are five principal factors dictating its potential hazard: (1)

T_p, (2) T_b; (3) T_e; (4) the body's affinity for the isotope; and (5) type e energy of decay products.

Elastic collision A collision between two particles is described as an elastic collision if neither of the particles absorbs energy internally. Although either of the particles may gain or lose energy during the collision, the sum of the kinetic energies of the participating particles remains unchanged as a result of the collision.

Elastic scattering Scattering effected through the agency of elastic collisions and therefore with conservation of kinetic energy of the system.

Electromagnetic radiation Electrical and magnetic energy in the form of waves of energy called photons, traveling through space at the speed of light. The spectrum of electromagnetic radiation ranges from long-wavelength, low-energy radio waves to very high-energy, short wavelength x-rays and γ-rays. In medicine, where x-rays from diagnostic equipment, γ-rays from Ir-192 the terms and photons from linear accelerators are used, they are all photons. The convention is that photons < 0.5 MeV from machines are x-rays and photons from isotopes are γ-rays, the high energies of ≥ 4 MeV from linear accelerators are known simply as photons. Also, when electrons are produced from isotopes, they are betas; however, from linear accelerators of sufficient energy, they are electrons. All energies are measured in electron volts (eV) and the $k = 1 \times 10^3$ so that a diagnostic x-ray may use 100 keV $= 100\ 000$ eV, and the $M = 1 \times 10^6$ for standard radiation oncology treatment, which ranges from 4 to 25 MeV $=$ 4 000 000–25 000 000 eV.

Electromagnetic spectrum The ordered array of known electromagnetic radiations, extending from the shortest cosmic rays, through γ-rays, x-rays, ultraviolet radiation, visible radiation, infrared radiation, including microwave and all other wavelengths of radio energy. The division of this continuum of wavelengths (or frequencies) into a number of named subportions is rather arbitrary, and with one or two exceptions, the boundaries of the several subportions are only vaguely defined. Nevertheless, characteristic types of physical systems capable of emitting radiation of those wavelengths correspond to each of the commonly identified subportions. Thus, γ-rays are emitted from the nuclei of atoms as they undergo any of several types of nuclear rearrangements; visible light is emitted, for the most part, by atoms whose planetary electrons are undergoing transitions to lower energy states; infrared radiations are associated with characteristic molecular vibrations and rotations; and radio waves, broadly speaking, are emitted by virtue of the accelerations of free electrons as, for example, the moving electrons in a radio antenna wire.

8

Electron A fundamental particle with a negative charge constituent of all atoms. Electrons take up most of the volume of the atom, but little of the mass. The mass of the electron is 9.11×10^{-28} g.

The term electron is also used collectively to include both the negative particle, also called negatron, and the positive particle of equal mass and charge, the positron. Both types may be emitted in β decay, but the lifetime of the positron is very short. The electrons in an atom occur in bound states around the central nucleus known as shells, denoted by the letters K, L, M, N, etc., corresponding to the quantum numbers n = 1, 2, 3, 4, etc; the total number of electrons permitted in each shell by the Pauli exclusion principle being $2n^2$ (i.e. 2 in the K-shell, 8 in the L-shell, etc.). The number of electrons is determined by the nuclear charge, which it must neutralize, and the electrons normally fill the shells from the lowest quantum number upwards. The electrons in the outer shell determine the chemical behavior of the atom. Beta particles, positrons, Auger, and internal conversion electrons have a range in tissue from a few micrometers to a few millimeters. However, the electron, in losing energy, follows a tortuous path and the mean range is typically a fifth of the maximum range. Energy losses are principally by excitation and ionization, but the interaction is less strong than for α particles because of the much smaller mass and single electronic charge. For example, a 1-MeV β particle creates about 20 ion pairs per mm at the start of its track and has linear energy transfer of 0.25 keV mm^{-1}. (An α particle of 5 MeV creates 700 ion pairs/mm.)

Electron capture Radioactive transformation in which an inner orbital electron is captured by an atom's nucleus. The capture of an electron by the nucleus leaves a vacancy in one of the inner electron shells. As a result, the product atom, and not the nucleus, has an energy above the ground state. This excess energy is lost either by the emission of the characteristic x-radiation of the daughter, or by the transfer of the excess energy to an outer electron, thereby ejecting it as an Auger electron. The x-rays and Auger electron have much lower energies than the particle emissions since the former result from extranuclear processes and the latter from intranuclear processes. Electron capture is more likely to occur than positron decay for nuclides with high Z in which the K shell is closer to the nucleus. Positron decay will be predominant at low Z provided that there is an energy difference of at least 1.02 MeV between the parent and daughter nuclides.

Electron volt (eV) The amount of energy gained by an electron in passing through a potential difference of 1 V. Larger multiple units of the electron volt are frequently used, viz, keV for thousand or kilo-electronvolts; MeV for millions or mega-electronvolts. 1 eV = 1.602×10^{-19} J. 1 eV = 1.602×10^{-12} erg. The joule (J) is the SI unit of energy.

Equivalent residual dose (ERD) The accumulated dose corrected or such physiological recovery as has occurred at a specific time. This is based on the ability of the body to recover to some degree from radiation injury following exposure. It is used only to predict immediate effects. It is used as an attempt to summate different types of radiation.

Erg A unit of energy corresponding to the work that is done when a force of 1 dyn produces a displacement of 1 cm in the direction of the force.

Exponential decay A decay process in which the decay decreases exponentially with time. The most common example of this process is the decay of activity of a radioactive substance with time, in accordance with the equation

$$A = A_o e^{-\lambda t}$$

where A and A_o are the activities present at times t and zero, respectively, and λ is the characteristic decay constant.

Exposure rate constant The exposure rate due to the emission of x- and γ-rays from a specific radionuclide of activity 1 Bq at a distance of 1 m. The 'exposure rate constant' replaced the former 'specific γ-ray constant', and has, in turn, been replaced by the 'air kerma-rate constant'. The term exposure rate constant has been retained, however, because adequate data in respect of the new quantity are not yet available.

Film badge A simple type of personnel radiation monitor that can be issued to individuals likely to be exposed to significant radiation doses. It consists of a metal or plastic case with a clip or pin for fastening to the outside of protective clothing, and holding a piece of photographic film (similar to that used for dental x-ray) wrapped in a light-tight envelope. Part of the film is covered by a thin metal screen. The unscreened portion is affected by β-, γ-, and x-rays, while the screened part containing a set of absorber filters is affected by the more energetic γ- and x-rays. When the film is developed, the blackening of the two parts due to radiation exposure enables an estimate to be made of the superficial and deep dose to which the wearer has been exposed. Films are usually issued for a fixed period such as a month, after which they are collected, processed, and radiation dose calculated with the aid of a densitometer by measuring the degree of blackening of the film. (A known dose causing exposure of the film is used to calibrate the densitometer.)

Free radical Any atom or molecule which possesses one unpaired electron. Such a radical usually exhibits considerable additive properties and high reactivity.

Gamma radiation (γ-radiation or γ-rays) Electromagnetic radiation of a short wavelength that is emitted by the nucleus of a radionuclide during radioactive decay. The wavelength of a γ-ray may be from 10^{-9} to 10^{-12} cm. Radioactive materials emit three types of radiation. The three types are called α-rays, β-rays, and γ-rays, respectively. Of the three radiations γ-rays are the most penetrating and require several inches of heavy material to reduce their intensity appreciably.

Gamma source A material from which γ-rays are emitted constitutes a γ-ray source. Generally, a γ-ray source refers to some radioactive material which emits γ-rays, in which case the γ-rays consist of discrete energy groups. However, the term is also applied to a source of bremsstrahlung, which is emitted in the passage of high-speed particles through matter. This source has a continuous energy distribution.

Geiger–Müller counter (G–M tube) A highly sensitive gas-filled tube with a collecting electrode (anode) maintained at high voltage to collect, multiply, and measure the ions produced by entering ionizing radiation. It is based upon the avalanche effect, which is observed when ions are accelerated by an electric field under appropriate conditions.

Genetic effects of radiation Inheritable changes (mutations) produced by the absorption of ionizing radiation. Mutations are abrupt changes in genes, the most characteristic feature of which is that the gene is permanently altered and handed down in the changed form, so that the character difference caused by the mutation is inherited. All ionizing radiations and also ultraviolet light have been found to cause mutation.

Gray (Gy) The SI unit is absorbed dose of ionizing radiation; 1 gray (Gy) = 1 J/kg = 100 rad.

Half-life ($T_{1/2}$) A unique characteristic of a radionuclide, defined by the time during which an initial activity of a radionuclide is reduced to one-half. It is related to the decay constant λ by $t_{1/2} = 0.693\lambda$. Half-lives may vary from less than a millionth of a second to millions of years, according to the isotope and element concerned. Biologic refers to the time for the body or an organ to eliminate one-half of the original material; physical refers to physical radioactive decay of nuclei to one-half their original numbers; effective refers to the combined effects of biological elimination and physical decay, which result in an observed half-life shorter than either of these two values individually. While the physical half-life cannot be altered, the biologic can be modified by formulating the isotope compound for more rapid elimination from the body.

Half-value layer (HVL) The thickness of any absorbing material required to reduce the intensity or exposure of a radiation beam to one-half of the initial value when placed in the path of the beam; synonym for half-thickness. This thickness 'T' may be related to the linear absorption coefficient μ by the equation $T = 0.693/\mu$.

Hardness A term referring to the penetrating power of x-rays. Soft x-rays, of lower frequency and hence lower energy, are less penetrating. Hard x-rays, having a higher frequency and greater energy, are more penetrating.

Incoherent scattering Scattering of photons of particles in which the scattering elements act independently of one another so that there are no definite phase relationships among the different parts of the scattered beam. The intensity of the scattered radiation at any point is obtained by adding the intensities of the scattered radiation reaching this point from the independent scattering elements.

Indirectly ionizing particles Undercharged particles or photons which can liberate directly ionizing particles or can initiate a nuclear transformation.

Inelastic collision A collision in which there are changes both in the internal energy of one or more of the colliding systems and in the sums of the kinetic energies of translation before and after collision.

Inelastic scattering Scattering effected by inelastic collisions, such as are involved in the Compton effect.

Inverse-square law Rule by which the radiation intensity of any source decreases inversely as the square of the distance between the source and the detector; RI = radiation intensity; D = distance:

$$RI = \frac{1}{D2}$$

Ion An atom or group of atoms bearing a positive (cation) or negative (anion) electric charge as a result of having lost or gained one or more electrons.

Ionization The process in which an atom or molecule separates into two parts (ions) which have opposite electrical charge. Two general types of ionization can be distinguished. First, there is that which occurs when a salt is dissolved in water and which results in the formation of two atomic or molecule ions in solution. Second, there is that which occurs when one or more electrons become detached from an atom or molecule.

Ionization of an atom or molecule requires that one or more electrons in the atom or molecule is raised from a bound to an unbound state. For an electron to become detached then, a certain minimum amount of energy, equal to the electron's binding energy, has to be transferred to the atom or molecule. This energy varies from element to element, ranging from about 5 eV for the alkali metals to about 20 eV for the rare gases.

The energy needs to produce ionization can be supplied when another particle collides with the atom or molecule. The colliding particle must in some way disturb the electrical field in the atom or molecule. For this reason suitable projectiles are other atoms, ions, γ-rays, and all the charged elementary particles. Other particles, like neutrons and neutrinos, produce negligible ionization because any electromagnetic interaction associated with them is very weak.

Ionization potential (E_i) The minimum energy needed to remove an outer ring electron from its orbit; 15 eV for atoms in the gaseous state.

Ionizing radiation Electromagnetic and particulate radiations may have sufficient energy to remove electrons from atoms (ionization). The energy of electromagnetic radiation is related to the frequency (or wavelength). Ionization of some atoms begins with rays of about 10 eV which corresponds to waves in the ultraviolet region. Thus, visible light (1 eV), microwaves (0.0001 eV), and lower frequencies may be considered to be non-ionizing. Ionization in human tissues is caused deliberately in radiotherapy using x-rays (0.1–10 MeV) and γ-rays (up to 100 MeV). Particulate radiation of β particles (electrons), α particles, neutrons, and heavy nuclei may be used. Visible light when reconfigured, i.e. laser can ionize.

Ion pair Two particles of opposite charge, usually referring to the electron and positive atomic or molecular residue resulting after the interaction of ionizing radiation with the orbital electrons of atoms.

Iridium-192 (Ir-192) $T\frac{1}{2} = 74.2$ days, γ-ray of 296–612 keV.

Isodose Descriptive of a locus at every point of which the absorbed dose is the same.

Isotope One of several nuclides having the same number of protons in their nuclei, and hence having the same atomic number, but differing in the number of neutrons, and therefore in the mass number. Almost identical chemical properties exist between isotopes of a particular element, for example, ^{11}C, ^{12}C, ^{13}C, ^{14}C are isotopes of carbon. The use of this term as a synonym for nuclide is not recommended. Nuclides are distinct nuclear species, while isotopes are nuclides of the same element.

Kerma Kinetic energy released in material. Non-stochastic quantity relevant only in the fields if indirectly ionizing radiations (photons or neutrons) or for any kerma is the expectation value of the energy transferred to charged particles per unit mass at a point of interest, including radiative loss energy but excluding energy passed from one charged particle to another.

Kerma can be expressed in units erg/g, rad, or J/kg. The latter unit is also the gray (Gy). The rad is still commonly employed for kerma and absorbed dose, but J/kg is preferred as it is an SI unit: $1 \text{ Gy} = 1 \text{ J/kg} = 10^2 \text{ rad} = 10^4 \text{ erg/g}$.

Kerma rate The kerma rate at a given point and time is expressed as J/kg·s (Gy/s) or in non-SI units erg/gs·s or rad/s, with other time units often substituted.

Lethal dose 50% (LD$_{50}$) Synonym for median lethal dose. Usually refers to whole body radiation and is the dose at which 50% of the subjects die.

Lethal dose 50/30 (LD$_{50/30}$) A dose of radiation (or other substance) which, when administered to a group of any living species, kills 50% of the group in 30 days. For CNS death, the higher the dose, the shorter the interval until death. At extremely high doses, death occurs during exposure from direct death of brain cells, meningitis, vasculitis, edema, and herniation. At even higher doses, death occurs in seconds. Thus, the LD$_{50}$/time period usually is set for different radiation syndromes, i.e. bone marrow, gastric, etc.

Lethal mutation A mutation that leads to the death of the individual who carries it, usually at an early stage of development. If recessive, the lethal mutation must be present in both the appropriate homologous chromosomes for its effects to be manifest.

Level A nucleus can possess only certain discrete amounts of internal energy. These values are those of the nuclear levels. The level with the least energy is termed the ground state. The energies of the other levels are usually given relative to it.

Lifetime The mean time between the appearance and disappearance (birth and death) of a particle. An excited state of an atom or nucleus also has a lifetime, which determines the rate at which it decays to another state.

Linear absorption coefficient Of a thin parallel beam of indirectly ionizing radiation passing through a uniform absorber, the fractional decrease of the beam's intensity per unit length of absorber traversed.

Linear accelerator Electrons can be accelerated to high velocities (up to 99% of the speed of light) in a straight wave guide driven by a microwave (e.g. 10 GHz) generator. Electrons are fed from a thermionic source into the evacuated wave guide, which contains a series of metal diaphragms with a hole in the middle so that with each wave the electrons move from one diaphragm to the next. The spacing of the diaphragms is increased down the length of the tube as the velocity of the electrons increases. At the far end they strike an x-ray target from which high-energy x-rays (6–25 MeV) are produced, or pass through a window to allow direct electron treatment. The resultant x-ray beam is attenuated by a beam-flattening filter, a circular piece of metal, thicker in the center than at the edge, which is introduced into the beam to produce a uniform x-ray intensity. The beam size is controlled by high metal collimators, which are adjustable over the range 4–40 cm. Beam intensity may be modified by a variety of metal filters, the most common being wedge shaped, which attenutate uniformly from one side of the beam to the other. Such devices are used in the treatment of deep cancers, since these high-energy rays have good penetration properties.

Linear attenuation coefficient The fractional number of photons removed from a beam of radiation per unit thickness of a material through which it is passing owing to all absorption and scattering processes.

Linear energy transfer (LET) Energy deposited by radiation per unit length of matter through which the radiation passes. Its usual unit is keV/μm.

Mass and weight The kilogram is the unit is mass. The word weight denotes a quantity of the same nature as a force; the weight of a body is the product of its mass and the acceleration due to gravity.

Mass attenuation coefficient (μm) For a given indirectly ionizing beam traversing a uniform medium, the ratio of the linear radiation absorption coefficient μ_1 and the density ρ of the medium ($\mu m - \mu_1/\rho$). The fractional decrease in radiation intensity per unit mass of medium traversed. Mass absorption coefficient.

Mass number (A) The mass number of a nuclide is the nearest integer to the actual or exact mass of a nucleus in atomic mass units (amu). There can be no ambiguity in this definition because the difference between the exact mass and the nearest integer is always very small. Since the exact masses of both the neutron and the proton in amu are both very close to unity, the mass number A gives the number of nucleons (neutrons and protons) in the nucleus.

Mass stopping power For a given material, the mass stopping power for charged particles can be written:

$$S/\rho = (1/\rho) \, (dE_s/d1)$$

where dE is the average energy lost by a charged particle of specific energy in traversing a path length $d1$, and ρ is the density of the medium.

Mean life The mean life of a radioactive substance is the average time for which its nuclei exist before disintegrating (symbol $= \tau$). It is the reciprocal of the disintegration constant (λ) and is equal to 1.442 times the half-life; $r = 1\lambda$.

15

Mean range The individual ranges in matter of heavy charged particles in a monoenergetic beam are not all the same; because of straggling, the individual ranges are spread about a mean range. Half the particles have ranges that exceed the mean range, and half have ranges that fall short of it.

Measurement of radioactivity A radioactive substance disintegrates with the emission of nuclear particles (α or β particles and/or photons—usually γ-rays), and the disintegration rate—which may be determined by measuring the rate of particle (or photon) emission—is decided by the amount of radioactive material present in the sample under investigation and by its half-life. Hence measurement of the emission rate provides a convenient method for the assay of such material.

Metastable state An unstable excited nuclear state having a finite and measurable half-life that decays to a more stable state by γ-emission without change in the atomic number; abbreviated by the letter m (e.g. ^{99m}Tc $\rightarrow$ ^{99}Tc). Also known as an isomeric state. (The prefix meta derives from the Greek work for 'almost.') In a quantum mechanical system such as a nucleus, the only truly stable state is the ground state of the system where the total energy has its minimum value. Most excited states decay very rapidly to the ground state by radiation and internal conversion and are said to be unstable.

Neutron Elementary nuclear particle with a mass approximately the same as that of a hydrogen atom and electrically neutral; its mass is 1.008986 mass units. Outside a nucleus a neutron is radioactive, decaying with a half-life of about 12 min to give a proton and an electron. Neutrons are commonly divided into subclassifications according to their energies as follows: thermal, around 0.025 eV; epithermal, 0.1–100 eV; slow $<$ 100 eV; intermediate, 102–105 eV; fast, $>$ 0.1 MeV. Since it has no charge it does not ionize and therefore has no fixed range in matter. It travels in a straight line until it is either scattered or absorbed by a nucleus. A neutron with very little kinetic energy can interact very strongly with a nucleus since it is not repelled electrostatically by the positive nuclear charge.

Neutron activation When certain materials are bombarded with neutrons, the nuclear reactions which take place lead to the production of radioactive nuclei. These products are frequently, but not necessarily, isotopes of the original nuclei.

Nuclear binding energy For a particle in a system, the net energy required to remove it from the system; for a system, the net energy required to decompose it into its constituent particles. Some of this represents the binding energy of orbital electrons, i.e. the energy required to strip the orbital electrons away from the nucleus. However, comparison of the total binding energy of a ^{12}C atom with the K-shell binding energy of carbon indicates that most of this energy is nuclear binding energy, i.e. energy required to separate the nucleons. When the mass of an atom is compared to the sum of the masses of its individual components (protons, neutrons, and electrons), it is always found to be less by some amount δm. This mass deficiency, expressed in energy units, is called the binding energy E_B of the atom.

$$E_B = \delta m c^2$$

Nuclear forces These are the strong short-range forces between nucleons that bind them together into nuclei.

Nuclear isomers Isotopes of elements having the same mass number and atomic number, but differing in radioactive properties such as half-life period.

Nucleon A common term for a constituent particle of the nucleus. This term commonly applies to protons and neutrons.

Nucleus The positively charged central portion of an atom comprising nearly all the atomic mass and consisting of protons and neutrons, except in hydrogen which consists of only one proton. It is about 10^{-12} cm in diameter. Only nuclei with an odd number of nucleons exhibit a net spin and therefore lend themselves to nuclear magnetic resonance (NMR) spectroscopy.

Nuclide The term nuclide indicates a species of atom having specified numbers of protons and neutrons in its nucleus. Nuclides of one and the same chemical element, i.e. nuclides with the same number of protons and differing only in the number of neutrons, are known as isotopes of the element concerned. Because of this, the term is often used erroneously as a synonym for 'isotope'. Isotopes are the various forms of a single element and therefore are a family of nuclides with the same number of protons. Nuclides are distinguished by their atomic mass and number as well as by energy state. Nuclides are distinct nuclear species, isotopes are nuclides of the same element. In some nuclides various energy states of the nucleus with finite lifetimes are possible. These states are called isomers of the nuclide. Isomeric nuclides have the same number of protons and neutrons and differ only in their energy content and thus their lifetime. The nature of a nuclide is indicated unambiguously by the chemical symbol of the element and the number of nucleons (sum of the protons (Z) and neutrons (N) = A, mass number) shown as an upper index to the left of the element symbol (e.g. ^{12}C, ^{32}P). Additionally, the number of protons (Z atomic number) can be given as a lower index on the left. Isomers in an excited, metastable state are indicated by an upper index 'm' (e.g. ^{99m}Tc). Approximately 1250 different nuclides are recognized at present, each being a distinct species of nucleus with its own characteristic nuclear properties. Of these, 280 are naturally occurring stable nuclides, while the remainder (radionuclides) undergo spontaneous radioactive decay with half-lives which vary from a fraction of a second to $> 10^{12}$ years. The only radionuclides which occur in nature are those with half-lives of the order of the age of the earth (or greater), or which are constantly being generated by natural nuclear processes.

Orbital electron An orbital electron is an electron in the extranuclear structure of the atom.

Paired production An absorption process for x- and γ-radiation in which the incident photon is annihilated in the vicinity of the nucleus of the absorbing atom with subsequent production of an electron and positron pair. This reaction only occurs for incident photon energies exceeding 1.02 MeV. This is an example of direct conversion of energy into matter according to Einstein's equation: $E = mc^2$. It only occurs when a γ-ray passes close to a nucleus, which appears to act as a catalyst for the process.

Parent A radionuclide that upon disintegration yields a specified nuclide, the daughter, either directly or as a later member of a radioactive series.

Phosphorus-32 (P-32) T½ = 14.3 days, β energy—1.7 MeV.

Photoelectric effect A process by which a photon ejects an electron from an atom. All the energy of the photon is absorbed in ejecting the electron and in imparting kinetic energy to it. A characteristic x-ray (or Auger electron) is subsequently produced when the vacated shell is filled by another orbital electron.

Photon A quantum of electromagnetic energy having no charge and characterized by its wavelength or frequency. Its energy content is the product of its frequency and Plank's constant, the equation for which is $E = h\nu$.

Physical half-life ($T_{1/2}$, T_p) The amount of time required for a radionuclide to reduce its radioactivity to one-half of its original value.

Primary ionization The ionization produced directly by the interaction of an energetic charged primary particle with the atoms of the matter through which it is passing, as contrasted with 'total ionization' which includes the 'secondary ionization' produced by δ-rays. In counter tubes: the total ionization produced by incident radiation without gas amplification.

Quality factor (Q) In radiation, a dimensionless variable weighting factor to be applied to the absorbed dose to provide an estimate of the relative human hazard of different types and energies of ionizing radiations. Values of Q are selected from experimental values of the Relative Biological Effectiveness

18

(RBE), which is the ratio of x- or γ-ray dose to that of the radiation in question giving the same kind and degree of biological effect. Q is chosen by the International Commission on Radiological Protection (ICRP) to be a smooth function of the unrestricted linear energy transfer (L∞) of the radiation. It is also called the collision stopping power.

Quality of radiation Penetration of radiation: frequently measured by its half-value layer (HVL). The HVL is the thickness of some standard material, which transmits 50% of the incident radiation.

Radioactive decay This is the spontaneous transformation with a measurable half-life of a nuclide into one or more different nuclides. The process involves the emission from the nucleus of α particles, electrons, positrons, γ-rays or the nuclear capture or ejection of orbital electrons, or fission. To be considered as radioactive, a process must have a measureable lifetime between about 10^{-10} and about 10^{17} years.

Radioactive equilibrium The condition in which the activities of the members of a radioactive chain decrease exponentially in time with the half-life of the chain precursor. Such radioactive equilibrium is only possible when the half-life of the precursor is longer than that of any other chain member. If the precursor half-life is so long that the change in the precursor population during the period of interest can be ignored, all the activities become sensibly equal, and the equilibrium is said to be secular; otherwise it is said to be transient.

^{90}Y/^{90}Sr is in secular equilibrium. Strontium-90 (Sr-90) has a half-life ($T\frac{1}{2}$) of 27.7 days and it decays to yttrium-90 (^{90}Y) and its principal β particle is 0.54 MeV. It is the ^{90}Y with a $T\frac{1}{2}$ of 64 days and a principal β^- (99.9%) with an energy of 2.274 MeV that is used for treatment. ^{90}Y alone can be used for treatment with replacement every 1–3 months (as the isotope decays, its dose rate increases leading to increasing treatment times). The Sr-90/Y-90 isotope has the advantage of the Sr-90 continuing to replenish the Y-90, so that decreases in dose rate are very slow.

Radiosensitivity The relative susceptibility of cells, tissues, organs, organisms, and any substances to the injurious action of ionizing radiation. Radioresistance and radiosensitivity are usually employed in a comparative sense, rather than in an absolute one.

Recoil electron An electron that has acquired its motion through a collision with another particle or through the emission of radiation.

Recoil nucleus A nucleus that has acquired its motion either through being struck by a nuclear particle or through the emission of radiation.

Recoil particle An particle that has acquired its motion through a collision with another particle or through the emission of radiation.

Relative biological effectiveness (RBE) An expression of the effectiveness of absorbed doses of different types of radiation, e.g. x-rays, neutrons, α particles. In general, the RBE may vary with the kind and degree of biologic effect considered, the duration of the exposure, and other factors. In general the higher the linear energy transfer (LET) of the radiation, i.e. the energy dissipated per unit distance along the track of an ionizing particle, the greater is the biological effect produced by a dose of 1 gray (Gy). Dense ionization, and hence LET, is associated with heavy particles (i.e. protons, deuterons, α particles, etc.), and these therefore tend to produce more biological effect per gray than x- and γ-rays, or electrons. The relative biological effectiveness of an ionizing radiation is defined as the dose of 250 kV x-radiation, which will produce the same biological effect as 1 Gy of the radiation in question. It should be emphasized that the RBE may have different values for the same radiation depending on the type of biological effect used as the criterion.

Roentgen equivalent man (rem) Non-SI unit of dose equivalent. The dose in rems is equal to the absorbed dose in rads multiplied by appropriate modifying factors aimed at expressing different types of radiation and different distributions to absorbed dose on a common scale related to the possible long-term radiation risks. For many radiations, including x, γ-, and β-radiation, and for most dose distributions, the modifying factor is unity and rems and rads are numerically equal. 1 rem = 0.01 sievert (Sv).

Scattered radiation Radiation that, through its interaction with matter, has undergone a change or changes in direction. In most cases radiation that has been scattered will have had its energy diminished.

Secular radioactive equilibrium In many cases radioactive nucleus is produced as a result of the decay of another and it is thus possible to have a chain of decay processes leading to successive radioactive products. When the life of the parent is very much longer than any of the products an equilibrium is reached, called secular radioactive equilibrium, in which case the number of atoms disintegrated per unit of time is the same for all products. Otherwise the equilibrium is referred to as transient.

Shell According to Pauli's exclusion principle the extranuclear electrons do not all circle around the nucleus in orbits of the same radius, but are arranged in orbits at various distances from the nucleus. The extranuclear orbital electrons are thus assumed to be arranged in a series of concentric spheres called shells, which are designated in the order of increasing distance from the nucleus as K, L, M, N, O, P, and Q-shells. The number of electrons that each of these shells can contain is limited. The electrons in the same shell are grouped into various subshells and all the electrons in the same subshell have the same orbital angular momentum.

Sievert (Sv) The SI unit of dose equivalent (J/kg). The absorbed dose in grays multiplied by the quality factor of the type of radiation. One Sievert = 100 rem.

SI units In 1948, the General Conference on Weights and Measures, a diplomatic conference responsible for the 'international unification and development of the metric system', instructed its International Committee for Weights and Measures to develop a set of rules for the units of measurement. The 'International System of Units' (Le Systeme International d'Unites, SI) was developed under this charge, adopted by the CGPM (Conference General des Poids et Measures) in 1960, and accepted by all signatories to the Meter Convention in 1977.

Source strength The strength of a radioactive source, meaning the amount of radioactive material contained in it, is expressed in curies or becquerels.

Specific activity The activity per unit mass of an element or compound containing a radioactive nuclide. The SI unit of specific activity is the becquerel per kilogram (Bq kg^{-1}) or becquerel per mole (Bq mol^{-1}). The non-SI unit is the curie per kilogram (Ci kg^{-1}) or curie per mole (Ci mol^{-1}).

Specific γ-ray constant For a nuclide emitting γ-rays: the product of exposure rate at a given distance from a point source of that nuclide and the square of that distance divided by the activity of the source, neglecting attenuation; it is expressed in SI units as C kg^{-1} m^2/MBq s (non-SI units: R cm^2/mCi h).

Stopping cross-section The linear stopping power (energy loss per unit thickness, dE/dx) divided by the number of atoms per unit volume of the stopping material.

Strontium Element symbol Sr, atomic number 38, atomic weight 87.62.

Teletherapy (From the Greek 'tele' meaning distant and 'therapia' meaning therapy). A radiotherapy method of using a radiation source in which the radioelement is shielded on all sides except one, thus giving a directional beam of radiation which is directed at a distant area to be treated.

Thin-window counter tube In order that radiation may be detected it must pass into the sensitive volume of the counter tube and produce ionization. In the case of short-range radiation, it is usual to provide the counter tube with a window through which the radiation may pass to penetrate into the sensitive volume. For the detection of α particles and soft β particles it is essential to use a thin window; counter tubes designed for this purpose are often referred to as thin-window counter tubes.

Tissue equivalent material Material which has the same reaction to radiation (e.g. absorption) as living tissue, and so can be used in models to study probable doses, radiation scatter, etc. Since soft tissue contains about 80% water, water itself is a very convenient tissue equivalent material for many purposes, e.g. phantoms in which to measure isodose curves. However, for other purposes such as the estimation of doses in irregularly shaped body sections, a solid material is more convenient. The main requirement is that the material has the same atomic number as soft tissue.

Xenon-133 (Xe-133) $T\frac{1}{2}$ = 5.3 days; principal γ-ray (37%) is 81 keV.

Yttrium Element symbol Y, atomic number 39, atomic weight 88.905.

2. ISOTOPES FOR USE IN VASCULAR BRACHYTHERAPY

Department of Medical Physics, Memorial Sloan–Kettering Cancer Center, New York, NY, USA

Howard I Amols

This chapter reviews the dosimetry of intraluminal irradiation of coronary and peripheral arteries using high activity gamma or beta seeds and wires in conjunction with balloon angioplasty; inflation of balloon catheters with radioactive liquid; and implantation of low activity radioactive stents. Isotope selection requires knowledge of the location and radiosensitivity of the target tissues, plus the radio-tolerance of normal tissues. Radiation dosimetry, safety, dose homogeneity, and practicality of source manufacture and delivery must all be considered. Unlike conventional brachytherapy, intravascular treatment of restenosis requires accurate knowledge of dose at distances of 0.5–5 mm from the radioactive source, which presents special calibration and treatment planning problems. More extensive discussion of these topics can be found in the literature.[1-4] The treatment volume is typically a 2–5-cm length of artery, 3–5 mm in diameter. Arterial wall thickness is typically 0.5–1.5 mm, but can be larger for diseased vessels. It is not known whether treatment of only the lumen wall is sufficient, or whether the media and adventitia must also be irradiated. Treatment doses of 8–20 Gy have been shown to be effective, but patient whole body dose, dose to normal vessels and myocardium, as well as dose to staff must be as low as possible.

Most catheter-based clinical trials to date have utilized one of three isotopes: Ir-192, Sr/Y-90, or P-32. Ir-192 is a relatively high-energy gamma-emitter and as such provides the best possible dose distribution to the target volume, but presents radiation safety problems because the high-energy gammas are difficult to shield. Sr/Y-90 and P-32 are all pure beta emitters which are easily shielded, although the limited range of the beta emissions results in more rapid dose fall off within the target volume than with Ir-192 gammas. Most radioactive stent trials have also utilized the beta emitter P-32. Another major difference between beta and gamma isotopes is the amount of activity required to achieve an adequate dose rate. For catheter-based treatments a dose rate of at least 1 Gy/min is desirable in order to keep treatment times under 30 min, and ideally under 10 min. This requires a minimum of 0.5–1.0 Ci activity for a high-energy gamma emitter such as Ir-192, with lower energy γ- or x-ray emitters (such as I-125 or Pd-103) requiring even higher activities (1–3 Ci). Beta emitters can deliver adequate dose rates with activities as low as 20–50 mCi. Radioactive stents on the other hand deliver their dose over the lifetime of the stent and require much lower amounts of activity—typically 1–10 µCi of P-32. Gamma stents (currently under development) may require activities of ⩾100 µCi.

More recently, other isotopes have been proposed and/or studied for possible use in intravascular brachytherapy. The search for alternatives to the above three isotopes is motivated by three factors:

1. Lower energy gammas (energy between 20 and 100 keV) produce dose distributions comparable to Ir-192, but are as easy to shield as beta sources.
2. Higher energy betas yield dose distributions superior to Sr/Y-90 and P-32 and are still easy to shield.
3. Other isotopes may permit alternate mechanisms for dose delivery such as liquid- or gas-filled radioactive balloons, liquid infusion, etc.

Table 2.1 lists some of the isotopes currently being used or considered for intravascular brachytherapy. The radial dose distribution and dose rate per curie are critical. It is assumed that any viable isotope can be fabricated into a

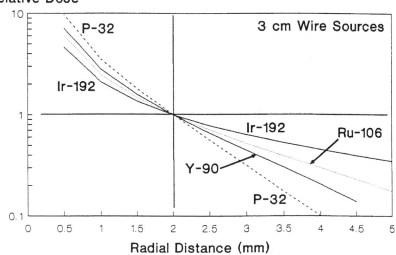

Figure 2.1 Radial dose vs distance for Ir-192, P-32, Sr/Y-90, and Ru-106 sources. Sources are 0.65 mm diameter × 30.0 mm length. Doses are normalized to 1.0 at a radial treatment distance of 2.0 mm. Doses for I-125 and Pd-103 are not plotted, but would be very similar to Ir-192.

Table 2.1 Possible isotopes for intraluminal brachytherapy

Isotope	Emission	Maximum energy (keV)	Average energy (keV)	Half-life	Comments
Ir-192	Gamma	612	375	74 days	Best dose distribution, hard to shield
I-125	X-ray	35	28	60 days	Good dose, easy to shield, needs high activity
Pd-103	X-ray	21	21	19 days	Good dose, easy to shield, needs high activity
P-32	Beta⁻	1710	690	14 days	Easy to shield, but dose penetration limited
Sr/Y-90	Beta⁻	2270	970	28 years	Better dose than P-32, but worse than gamma
Y-90	Beta	2270	970	64 h	Identical to Sr/Y-90, but shorter half-life
W/Re-188	Beta⁻	2130	780	69 days	Similar dose to Y-90; possible wire source
Re-188	Beta⁻	2130	780	69 days	Similar dose to Y-90; used for liquid balloons
V-48	Beta⁺	690	230	6 days	Possible use for radioactive stent
Xe-133	Beta⁻	340	113	5.3 days	Prototype gas-filled balloon
Tc-99m	Gamma	140	140	6 h	Prototype liquid infusion catheter
X-ray tube	X-ray	30	10	Not applicable	Prototype x-ray tube for catheter use
Ru/Rh-106	Beta⁻	3540	1180	1 year	Higher energy beta, hard to produce

0.65-mm diameter by 30-mm length source. Figure 2.1 presents relative dose vs radial distance (normalized at a distance of 2 mm) for several isotopes. All sources show rapid dose fall off vs distance with betas having greater fall off than gammas because of the short range of low-energy electrons. Note that for electon sources, increasing the energy of the source has a great impact on the dose penetration and dose fall off, but for gammas the dose distributions are almost identical for any source with energy > 20–30 keV.

Because of radiation safety concerns regarding gammas, efforts have been directed towards developing new beta sources. P-32 is a pure β^-/emitter with transition energy of 1.71 MeV. Sr-Y is a 'parent-daughter' pair of pure β^-/emitters with transition energies of 0.540 and 2.27 MeV respectively. Y-90 can be used alone (half-life 64 h), or in radioactive equilibrium with Sr-90 (half-life 28 years). W/Re is another parent-daughter pair of β^-/emitters with transition energies of 0.430, and 2.13 MeV respectively. Re-188 can be used alone as a liquid source (half-life 17 h) or W/Re can be used as a wire source with a half-life of 69 days. Re-188 and Y-90 have similar dose distributions. So-called parent-daughter isotopes are a convenient way of combining the advantages of a high-energy beta (typically the daughter isotope) and a long half-life (typically the parent isotope).

Dose uniformity to the arterial wall depends on source centering and the cylindrical symmetry of the artery. Centering errors as small as 0.5 mm in a 3-mm diameter vessel result in dose asymmetries ranging from 2.6 for Ir-192 to 3.0 for P-32. Dose uniformity can be improved by the use of centering catheters. An alternate approach is to inflate the balloon catheter with a radioactive liquid or gas that automatically centers the source within the lumen. Concentrations > 60 mCi/ml yield acceptable dose rates for liquids, and such concentrations are achievable for Re-188. The use of radioactive impregnated stents has the advantage of intimate contact with the vessel walls and automatic centering, and requires very low activities (several μCi of beta emitter). The dose distribution from stents, however, will not be uniform because of the gridded structure of the stent, and the resulting non-homogeneous distribution of radioactivity. β^- (such as P-32), β^+ (such as V-48), or low-energy x-ray (such as Pd-103) emitters can be used in stents.

The success of treatment will depend on delivering an adequate dose to target tissues (8–20 Gy) while limiting the normal tissue dose to 30–45 Gy. If the target tissues are confined to the lumen wall then radiation dose penetration from betas may be sufficient and their advantageous safety aspects may prove superior. If the target is deeper in the media or adventitia then the superior dose fall off of gammas may prove advantageous. Dosimetry, source design, and treatment planning thus remain difficult problems for endovascular brachytherapy. Short treatment distances and large dose gradients make accurate measurements of in vivo doses virtually impossible—most traditional dosimeters are too large to be of value in such measurements. Development of an optimal source is difficult because of the high activities and small volumes required. None of the currently available gamma or beta sources is truly ideal. Gamma sources present significant radiation safety problems, and beta sources may not have significant range to treat all types of lesions.

References

1. Amols HI, Zaider M, Weinberger J et al. Dosimetric considerations for catheter based beta and gamma emitters in the therapy of neointimal hyperplasia in human coronary arteries. *Int J Radiat Oncol Biol Phys* 1996; **36**:913–921.

2. Amols HI. Review of endovascular brachytherapy physics for prevention of restenosis. *Cardiovascular Radiation Medicine* 1999; **1**:64–71.

3. Amols HI, Reinstein LE, Weinberger J. Dosimetry of a radioactive coronary balloon dilation catheter for treatment of neointimal hyperplasia. *Med Phys* 1996; **23**:1783–1788.

4. Nath R, Amols HI, Coffey C et al. Intravascular brachytherapy physics: report of the AAPM radiation therapy task group no. 60. *Med Phys* 1999; **26**:119–152.

3. GLOSSARY OF RADIATION PHYSICS FOR VASCULAR RADIATION THERAPY

Ionizing Radiation Division, Physics Laboratory, National Institute of Standards and Technology, Gaithersburg, MD, USA

Bert M Coursey, Stephen M Seltzer, Christopher G Soares and Brian E Zimmerman

Radioactive sources of beta-particle and gamma-ray emitting radionuclides are under investigation for use in intravascular brachytherapy. This interdisciplinary field draws on experimental and theoretical nuclear and medical physics.

Physics of radioactive decay and radiation interactions

Radioactivity is the phenomenon of emissions of neutral or charged particles, or electromagnetic radiations from unstable atomic nuclei (**radionuclides**). Radioactivity is the amount of a radionuclide in a particular energy state at a given time. Mathematically, it is defined as the quotient of dN by dt, where dN is the number of spontaneous nuclear transformations from that energy state in the time interval dt.

The unit of activity in the international system (SI) of units is the **becquerel** (Bq), which has the unit reciprocal second (s^{-1}). In many fields the older unit, the **curie** (Ci), is still in use, where 1 Ci = 3.7×10^{10} Bq (exactly).

The activity of an amount of radionuclide is given by the product of the **decay constant**, λ, and the number N of nuclei present, thus $A = \lambda N$.

The **half-life** is the time necessary for one-half of the nuclei to decay. The activity at any time t can be computed using the initial activity A_0 and the decay time t according to the equation

$$A = A_0 \exp(-\lambda t) = A_0 \exp(-0.69315 \, t/T_{1/2}).$$

Beta particles are high-energy electrons emitted by nuclei that contain too many or too few neutrons. For a system with excess neutrons, the neutron is transformed into a proton, and in the process an electron and an antineutrino are emitted.

The emitted negatively charged beta particles, usually denoted as β^-, have a continuum of energies from zero to a maximum energy denoted by E_β max.

Positrons are positively charged electrons (antiparticles of the electron) emitted by the nucleus. They are usually denoted as β^+ and have an energy distribution somewhat similar to that of β^- emitters.

Gamma rays are photons emitted during nuclear de-excitation processes. These γ-ray transitions may be from a metastable excited state, or between levels in a daughter nucleus. The large majority of γ-rays from fission-product and man-made radionuclides have energies between 20 keV and 2 MeV.

X-rays are photons emitted during atomic relaxation processes. X-rays are often emitted from radionuclides because orbital electrons can be involved in the nuclear transformation process. In the **electron capture** process, for example, the nucleus captures an electron (usually a K-shell electron, since it is closer to the nucleus), and a proton and electron form a neutron. This process leaves a K-shell vacancy, and a characteristic x-ray from the daughter nucleus can be emitted, as orbital electrons from higher shells fill the vacancy.

Annihilation radiation is a form of photon radiation associated with a class of radioactive decays. Positrons, since they are antiparticles of ordinary electrons, cannot survive long in normal matter. Thus, positrons emitted during radioactive decay will slow down in matter usually until they reach thermal equilibrium. They combine with an electron in an annihilation event in which their combined mass (1.022 MeV) is converted to energy. This takes the form of two annihilation quanta of 0.511 MeV each, which are oppositely directed (to ensure the conservation of momentum).

Bremsstrahlung is the photon radiation emitted by the deceleration of an electron in the Coulomb field of an atom. Thus, bremsstrahlung radiation is present during all beta decay processes since the emitted beta particles (both negatrons and positrons) slow down in matter; it has a continuum of photon energies extending up to the maximum beta-particle energy.

Electromagnetic radiation (γ-ray and x-ray photons) interacts with matter principally by three processes: photoelectric absorption, Compton scattering and pair production.

In the **photoelectric process**, which dominates at lower energies, the photon transfers its energy to an atomic electron, which is then ejected from the atom with an energy equal to that of the incident photon minus the electron's binding energy.

In **Compton scattering** (incoherent scattering), the photon loses a fraction of its energy to an atomic electron, and a scattered secondary photon emerges — generally in a direction different from that of the incident photon. Higher energy photons will undergo multiple Compton scatter events until the process is finally terminated by a photoelectric absorption.

For photons with energies exeeding 1.022 MeV, the process of **pair production** can occur, whereby an electron–positron pair is formed. The

positron produced will ultimately annihilate with the production of two
0.511-MeV photons (or in flight). The three interaction processes compete as
a function of photon energy, electron density, and nuclear charge of the
stopping material.

Quantitative measures of the photon interactions in matter are
attenuation coefficients based on **cross-sections** for specific
interactions. The total, **narrow-beam attenuation coefficient** μ is given
by the sum $\mu = \mu_{\text{photoelectric}} + \mu_{\text{Compton}} + \mu_{\text{pair production}}$. The attenuation process
for a beam of photons traversing a slab of matter is an exponential function
of the form

$$I = I_0 \exp(-\mu x)$$

where I and I_0 are the intensities of the transmitted beam and the incident
beam, respectively; x is the distance traveled in matter, and μ is the linear
attenuation coefficient. A useful procedure is to express distances in terms of
the mass thickness — the product of density ρ and thickness x. The beam
transmission equation can then be rewritten as

$$I = I_0 \exp[(-\mu/\rho)(\rho x)]$$

where μ/ρ is called the **mass attenuation coefficient**, which in contrast
to the linear attenuation coefficient does not depend on the density of the
absorber, but only on its composition.

The two quantitative parameters used to describe the interaction of beta
particles as they slow down in matter are stopping power and range.

Total mass stopping power, S/ρ, is the quotient of dE by ρdx, where
dE is the energy lost by a charged particle in traversing a distance dx in the
material of density ρ. For energies for which the nuclear interactions can be
neglected, the total mass stopping power can be represented as the sum of a
collisional term and a radiative term

$$S/\rho = 1/\rho \cdot (dE/dx)_{\text{col}} + 1/\rho \cdot (dE/dx)_{\text{rad}}.$$

Range for electrons of a given energy in a material is an important
parameter in designing intravascular radiation sources. Although an electron
does not travel in a straight line as it slows down, a useful parameter is the
mean total path length traveled, which is given by

$$r_0 = \int_0^E \rho/S \, dE$$

where E is the incident electron energy.

Experimental radiation dosimetry

Most of the experimental techniques in use for intravascular radiation therapy were originally developed for use in brachytherapy for radiation oncology. These are described in the bibliography. The major difference, from an experimental point of view, is that reference distances in oncology are measured in centimeters, whereas for intravascular therapy they are measured in millimeters. This puts a greater requirement on the spatial resolution of the detector.

Absorbed dose is the quantity of main interest to the clinician for both beta and gamma sources. It is the quotient of dE by dm, i.e. the differential energy absorbed in the differential mass in the medium. The unit of absorbed dose is the **gray** (Gy), which is 1 joule per kilogram.

Depth dose defines the relationship between the absorbed dose and depth in the medium. Thus, one can define a reference depth in terms of the absorbed dose at 2 mm from the center of the center line of the source.

Air kerma strength is the quantity used to specify the strength of a gamma-ray emitting radionuclide. Kerma, <u>k</u>inetic <u>e</u>nergy <u>r</u>eleased per unit <u>m</u>ass, is a measure of the energy released in a volume of air at some distance from a radioactive source. For photon-emitting sources used in brachytherapy it has units of Gy s^{-1} m^2.

Ionization chambers are the class of radiation detectors in which the radiation produces ionization events in a gas. The gas is contained in a chamber equipped with two electrodes which differ in potential by several hundred to a thousand volts. Ion pairs formed by the incident radiation travel to the positively and negatively charged electrodes. The charge collected (or current) is a measure of the radiation field. **In-air ionization chambers** are chambers that communicate with the air. Therefore, humidity, pressure and temperature corrections must be applied. They are widely used for high-activity sources, such as high dose rate iridium-192 sources.

Extrapolation chamber is a primary standard chamber used to establish the absorbed dose rate for beta-particle-emitting sources. A variable volume ionization chamber is used and the quotient dI/dx, where I is the chamber current and x is the distance separating the electrodes, is extrapolated to zero distance.

Well ionization chambers are sealed, pressurized ionization chambers (also called dose calibrators), which are intended for use in assaying brachytherapy sources. Their response must be determined for each source type and will in general depend on the particular source jig and catheter used for the measurement.

Scintillation detectors are made of material that absorb ionizing radiation and convert a fraction of the energy into light. These photons are transmitted by lightguides to photodetectors, which include diodes and photomultiplier tubes.

Thermoluminescent dosimeters (TLD) are based on inorganic materials which store a fraction of the energy deposited by a radiation field. The stored energy may be released by heating the TLD with a thermal source or a laser. Traditional TLDs are too large for use with intravascular therapy seeds, but sheets of material are now available with pixel sizes of 100 µm.

Radiochromic films consist of a thin emulsion on a mylar backing in which a chemical detector produces a blue color which is proportional to the amount of radiation received. These films are widely used to measure autoradiographs of seeds used in intravascular brachytherapy. With proper calibration they can also be used to establish the **absorbed dose** in a **phantom** material.

Phantom is the material used for the absorbing medium in the experimental dose measurement. Several different phantom materials are used in intravascular therapy including **water phantoms** and those fabricated from plastics (**A-150 plastic, tissue-equivalent plastic, solid water**).

Theoretical radiation dosimetry

Both theoretical and computational methods in radiation dosimetry have advanced rapidly over the past two decades. At this point in the development of intravascular radiation therapy, they are indispensable tools for seed designers and clinical investigators. The ability to predict the depth–dose relationship in a variety of arteries, with different materials (blood, calcifications, smooth muscle cells, etc), for many radionuclides, and in many configurations (catheters, stents, marker seeds) dictates the use of computational methods in conjunction with experiments to establish the basic dosimetry. Some of the main tools are listed here.

Emitted spectrum is the beta-particle energy distribution for a given radionuclide. This distribution must be taken into account in a theoretical dose calculation.

Monte Carlo methods are computer models based on 'chance', i.e. dictated by known probability distributions. A geometry is defined comprising a source and detector medium. Electron and/or photon histories are 'emitted' from the source and then 'followed' and 'scored' as the radiation undergoes interactions in the medium. Since it is a statistical process, a large number of histories are followed. The accuracy of the calculation will depend on the completeness and accuracy of the modeling employed, and its applicability requires a detailed specification of the source geometry and the medium (lumen, catheter, tissue).

ETRAN is a general-purpose coupled electron–photon Monte Carlo transport code developed at the National Institute of Standards and Technology (NIST). A related code is the **ITS** code developed at Sandia National Laboratory, which is a more general and user-friendly code for intravascular radiation therapy calculations.

MCNP is a Monte Carlo code developed at Los Alamos National Laboratory, which was originally intended for neutrons and gamma rays, but has been extended to include electrons as well, through the incorporation of ITS algorithms.

EGS is a coupled electron–photon Monte Carlo code originally developed at Stanford University and more recently extended to a variety of applications in medical physics.

Point kernels for photons or electrons give the dose distribution from a point source in a homogeneous medium such as water. Extended source and absorbing media configurations are treated by superpositions of point kernels using integration algorithms. Such calculations are much faster than Monte Carlo methods but are inherently approximate.

4. GLOSSARY OF RADIOBIOLOGICAL TERMINOLOGY OF RELEVANCE TO VASCULAR BRACHYTHERAPY

Center for Radiological Research, Columbia University, New York, NY, USA

David J Brenner

Absorbed dose	The mean energy imparted by ionizing radiation to matter in a given volume divided by the mass of the matter in that volume. The unit of absorbed dose is the gray (Gy).
Accelerated repopulation	Increase in the rate of cell division, often caused by a radiation exposure.
Acute exposure	A dose given in a short period of time — typically not more than a few minutes.
Alpha:beta ratio	The ratio of the parameters α and β in the equation describing the shape of the survival curve or the isoeffect plot (if the ratio is large, the sensitivity to changes in fractionation is low).
Apoptosis	Mode of cell death characterized by nuclear fragmentation, cell lysis, and phagocytosis by neighboring cells.
Becquerel (Bq)	The becquerel is a unit of activity used to measure the amount of radioactive disintegrations per unit time. One Bq is one transformation in 1 second. There are 3.7×10^{10} Bq in 1 curie (Ci).
Beta particles	High-speed electrons that are emitted from the nucleus of an atom.
Brachytherapy	Radiation therapy with a radioactive source placed in or near the target cells.
Cell killing	Inability of cells to replicate.
Chronic exposure	Dose of radiation delivered over a prolonged period of time.
Clonogen	Cell capable of producing a clone of genetically identical progeny.
Dose rate	Dose per unit time.
Dose rate effect	Change in the effectiveness of a given dose caused by changes in dose rate. Effectiveness usually decreases with decreasing dose rate, owing to repair of sublethal damage.

Doubling time	Time taken for a cell population to double its size.
Early effects	Sequelae from a radiation treatment which is manifest during or within a few days of the treatment.
Effective dose	The sum over specified tissues of the product of the equivalent dose in tissue (H_T) and the weighting dose for that tissue (w_T), i.e. $E = \Sigma\ w_T \cdot H_T$.
Equivalent dose (HT)	A quantity used for radiation protection purposes that takes into account the different probability of effects which occur from the same dose delivered by radiations with different biological effectiveness. It is the product of the average dose in a specified organ or tissue (D_T) and the radiation weighting factor (w_R). The unit of equivalent dose is joules per kilogram ($J\ kg^{-1}$) and its special name is the sievert (Sv).
External beam irradiation	Radiation therapy from a radiation source located outside the body, often an accelerator.
Fractionation	Splitting up of a radiation treatment into multiple smaller treatments, typically to spare normal tissues.
Gamma rays	High-energy electromagnetic waves or photons emitted from the nucleus of an atom.
Genetic effects	Effects from some agent that are seen in the offspring of the individual who received the agent. The agent would be encountered preconception.
Gray (Gy)	The special name for the unit of absorbed dose; $1\ Gy = 1\ J\ kg^{-1}$.
Growth delay	Extra time required for an irradiated versus an unirradiated group of cells to reach a given size.
Growth fraction	The proportion of cells that are in cycle in a population of cells.
Ionizing radiation	Radiation with enough energy so that, during an interaction with an atom, it can remove tightly bound electrons from their orbits, causing the atom to become charged or ionized. Examples are γ-rays, x-rays, β particles, α-rays, and neutrons.
Late effects	Sequelae to a radiation exposure which is manifest some time after the completion of treatment.
Linear–quadratic (LQ) model	Model in which the effect (E) is a linear–quadratic function of dose (D), i.e. $E = \alpha D + \beta D^2$. Used to predict isoeffect doses between different treatments.
Low dose rate	Delivery of radiation chronically over a time typically significantly longer than 1 hour. In principle allows the greatest differential in effects between early and late responding tissues.

Mitotic cell death	Cell death caused by failure to complete mitosis correctly and produce two viable daughter cells.
Negligible individual dose (NID)	A level of effective dose that can be dismissed as insignificant. The NID is currently 0.01 mSv/year.
Non-ionizing radiation	Radiation without enough energy to remove tightly bound electrons from their orbits around atoms. Examples are microwaves and visible light.
Organ or tissue weighting factor (w_T)	A factor that indicates the ratio of the risk of stochastic effects attributable to irradiation of a given organ or tissue (T) to the total risk when the whole body is uniformly irradiated.
Radiation	Energy transmitted in the form of high-speed particles or electromagnetic waves. Examples are visible light, radio and television waves, ultraviolet, and microwaves. These examples are of non-ionizing radiation because they do not carry enough energy to remove electrons from atoms.
Radiation weighting factor (w_R)	A factor used for radiation protection purposes that accounts for differences in biological effectiveness between different radiations. The radiation weighting factor (w_R) is independent of the tissue weighting factor (w_T).
Radioactivity	The spontaneous transformation of an unstable atom, resulting in the emission of radiation. This process is referred to as a transformation, a decay, or a disintegration of an atom.
Redistribution	Gradual synchronization of cells into the same part of the cell cycle, during treatment, as sensitive cells are preferentially killed.
Repair of sublethal damage	Repair of non-lethal injury, such as a DNA double strand break.
Senescence	Inability of the progeny of cells to undergo unlimited divisions.
Sievert (Sv)	The special name for the unit of effective dose and equivalent dose, 1 Sv = 1 J kg^{-1}.
Somatic effects	Effects from some agent, such as radiation, that are seen in the body of the individual who receives the agent.
Stochastic effects	Effects in which the probability, rather than the severity, is a function of radiation dose without threshold.

Sublethal damage	Non-lethal injury, such as a DNA double-strand break, that can be repaired or can accumulate with further dose to become lethal.
Teratogenic effects	Effects from some agent that are seen in the offspring of the individual who received the agent. The agent must be encountered during the gestation period.
Volume effect	The dependence of the biological effect on the size of the irradiated area. Typically irradiation of larger volumes produces more biological damage per unit dose.
X-rays	High-energy electromagnetic waves or photons not emitted from the nucleus, but normally emitted by energy changes in atomic electrons.

5. PRINCIPLES OF REMOTE AFTERLOADERS

Radiation Oncology, New York Presbyterian Hospital (Cornell), New York, NY, USA

Suhrid Parikh and Dattatreyudu Nori

Definition	The basic concept of 'afterloading' involves the following—'unloaded' tubes or applicators are inserted into the target volume to be irradiated. These are subsequently 'loaded' with the radioactive source (hence the term 'afterloading'). In the early days of radiotherapy this afterloading was performed manually. Today, the radioactive sources are stored in a shielded container, and inserted into the tubes or applicators via a remotely controlled afterloading device—hence the term 'remote afterloading'.

History	• The earliest afterloaders were manually operated; an operator stood behind a lead screen and moved the iridium-192 (Ir-192) sources to and from the applicator tubes in the patient • The first high dose-rate (HDR) remote afterloader with a mechanical control of the source movement was developed at the Memorial Hospital in 1964 by Henschke and colleagues • The first commercial HDR remote afterload was developed in 1964 and marketed by the Atomic Energy of Canada Ltd under the name of Brachytron

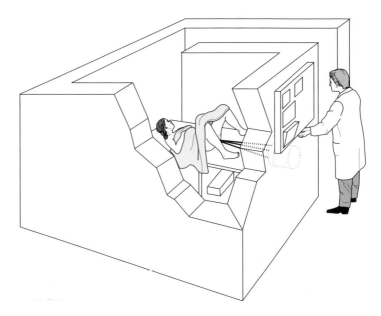

Figure 5.1 *Schematic layout of a high dose-rate brachytherapy suite.*

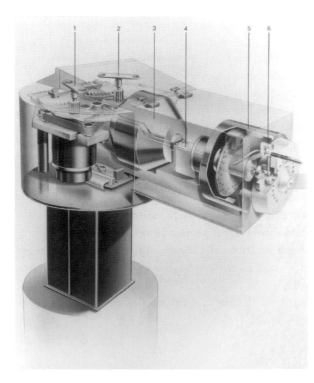

Figure 5.2
Components of an HDR
unit.
1 Source cable drive
2 Check cable drive
3 Safe for the source
4 Automatic calibration
5 Indexer
6 Optical verification
of applicator
connection
(Reproduced with the
kind permission of
Nucletron, Inc.)

Common features of most HDR units (Figures 5.1 and 5.2)

- The *HDR unit* consists of a mobile base that supports an enclosure for the necessary electrical components along with the source safe. Units typically weigh 100–250 kg and have an area of 1.5 m^2. The source safe is made of tungsten or depleted uranium and houses one or two 10.0 or 12.0 Ci sources.

- The *source drive mechanism* consists of a stepping motor which moves the source in a few seconds from the safe to the applicator; then, under computer control, it moves the source through the applicator in a precise fashion, stopping for a variable amount of time ('dwell time') at different points along the applicator ('dwell positions').

- The source drive mechanism is connected to the applicators via *transfer tubes (source-guide tubes)*. Generally, HDR units have self-testing mechanisms to test applicator connectors. If the applicator connector fails, the source will not leave the unit or will automatically retract back into it.

- Iridium-192 is generally used as the *source*, owing to its very high specific activity of 400 Ci/g. This allows the source to be as small as 0.6–1.0 mm in diameter. One or more such cylinders or pellets of radioactive material are sealed inside a thin-walled metal *source capsule* designed to absorb any undesired β-rays. The diameter of the capsule is critical because the clinical situation may limit the size of the applicator tube that can be inserted into tissues, while the length of the capsule determines how acute a curve the source can negotiate.

- The source capsule is welded to a *source drive cable*, which is driven by the source drive mechanism. It extends the source out of, and away from the machine; typical distances vary from 900 mm to 1500 mm.

- There is also a *simulated (dummy) source or cable* used to check the whole system and the source path; if the dummy cannot successfully negotiate the system, the real source cannot be used.

- The *remote control unit* stands outside the treatment vault and is usually a dedicated microprocessor that controls the HDR unit and the source movement. The information from the treatment planning computer (regarding the various dwell positions and the dwell times at each of these positions) is directly transferred to the control unit either via a serial cable or via programming cards.

- Specific features of selected HDR remote afterloaders are outlined in Table 5.1.

Table 5.1 Specific features of selected HDR remote afterloaders

Features	microSelectron (HDR) Nucletron Engineering BV (Netherlands)	Curietron 192 Oris (CIS-US) (France)	GammaMed 12i ISOTOPEN–TECHNIK DR. Sauerwein Gmbh (Germany)	VariSource Varian, Inc. (USA)
Number of sources	1 × 10 curie, ^{192}Ir	2 × 10 curie, ^{192}Ir	1 × 20 curie, ^{192}Ir	1 × 12 curie, ^{192}Ir
Physical size (capsule)	1.1 mm outer diameter × 5.0 mm length	1.2 mm outer diameter × 14 mm length	1.1 mm outer diameter × 6.5 mm length	0.59 mm outer diameter × 10 mm length
Smallest outer diameter of applicators	1.4 mm	4.7 mm	1.6 mm	0.89 mm
Method of source attachment	Source laser welded to drive cable	Source silver soldered to steel drive cable	Source welded to steel cable	Source permanently connected to platinum wire
Maximum source extension	1500 mm	1500 mm	1250 mm	1500 mm
Number of applicator channels	18	20	24	10

Method of source movement	Step forward; 48 steps of 2.5 mm over 120 mm length; 5 mm over 240 mm	Step forward; 30 steps over the last 800 mm of the catheter	Step back; 40 steps to 400 mm length; 1 mm to 10 mm steps	Step back in 11-mm increments over 200 mm
Source arrangements and dose calculations	Point source at 48 positions, 2.5 mm apart, dwell time to 999 s, in increments of 0.1 s	Point source at 30 positions, dwell times from 1 s to 999.9 s	Stepping source and dwell times to 999 s in 1-s increments	Step/dwell times used to achieve desired dose distribution
Method of source retraction in the event of failure	Dual monitors and backup battery; emergency hand crank	Backup battery and winch	Hand crank; backup battery	Backup battery; mechanical crank
Control unit and isodose planning system	Separate control unit and isodose planning system	Separate control unit and isodose planning system	Integral control unit and isodose planning system	Integrated control unit and isodose planning system
Dose optimization	Yes, 300 optimization points	Yes	Yes, 60 optimization points	Yes
Special features	Memory storage — 99 standard treatments	Can use two sources simultaneously	Memory storage of all planned and treated patients	Small source size; allows use of 20-gauge interstitial needles

Outline of an HDR treatment procedure

Following the insertion of the applicators into the target volume, simulation x-rays are obtained with dummy wires placed within the applicators. The dummy wires have radiopaque markers along them at 1-cm intervals. The desired volume to be treated is marked on the x-ray by the radiation oncologist, and this volume is digitized into a treatment planning computer. The actual dose and prescription point is decided. With this information, and the help of an optimization program, the optimal dwell positions and dwell times at each position, along the applicator can be determined. This information is transferred to the remote control unit to regulate the source movements. The applicators are then connected to the HDR unit and the treatment is delivered. Throughout the treatment, the patient and the HDR unit are monitored from outside the treatment vault by remotely operated video cameras, and there is an arrangement for two-way communication between the patient and the treating personnel.

General advantages of high dose-rate brachytherapy

- *Short treatment time*—this ensures that the blood flow in the vessel is compromised only for a brief period of time (2–5 min), even with a centering device.
- *Single stepping source* (instead of a fixed length source train)—allows personnel to treat the precise length of the vessel required. With fixed length sources, there is always the potential for under- or over-treating, since the number of source lengths available at a given time is limited.
- *Ability to optimize the dose distribution*, by varying the dwell times at different points along the vessel. This allows personnel to ensure that the ends of the target volume are adequately covered (to achieve this with a source train would require differential loading, with higher activities at the ends, or a longer length would have to be treated (Figures 5.3 and 5.4).
- *Radiation protection*—this approach is associated with the least radiation exposure to all the treating personnel, since the entire radiation therapy is delivered in a shielded room.
- *Cost-effective*—the HDR approach involves the use of a brachytherapy system that is already in place in the radiation oncology department. There is no additional expense for special source trains, nor is there any extra work on the part of the physicists (in terms of source calibration, handling, storage, inventory control, source disposal, etc).

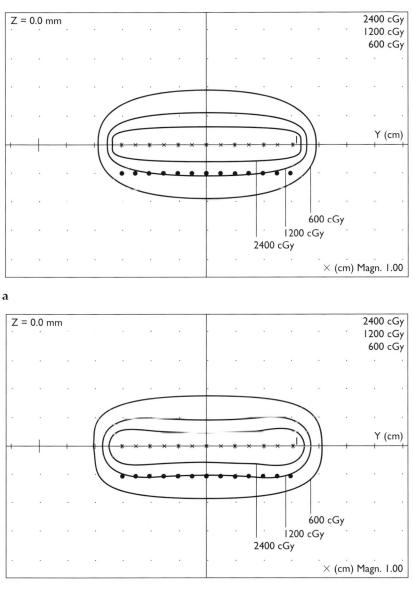

Figure 5.3 *Dose distributions showing the need for optimization to ensure that the ends of the target do not get underdosed. (a) Non-optimized distribution with equal dwell times of the source at each position. The circles represent the target volume. Note that the two circles at either end are not encompassed by the 1200 cGy curve, and are being underdosed (so-called 'edge effect'). (b) The same target with an optimized distribution, such that the dwell times of the source at either end are increased. Note how all the circles are encompassed by the 1200 cGy isodose.*

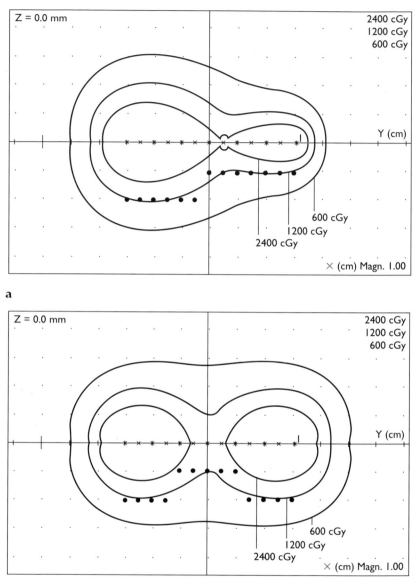

Figure 5.4 *(a) and (b) are examples of how the dose distribution can be shaped to encompass any given target volume.*

Indications for clinical use

- High dose-rate intracavity brachytherapy for a variety of malignancies, including cervical and endometrial carcinoma, bronchogenic and esophageal carcinomas, carcinoma of the biliary tree, anorectal carcinomas, nasopharyngeal carcinomas, etc (Figure 5.5)
- HDR interstitial brachytherapy for solid tumor masses, including head and neck malignancies, gynecologic cancers, etc
- HDR brachytherapy using surface molds in a variety of innovative settings
- HDR endovascular brachytherapy to prevent post-angioplasty restenosis (under evaluation)

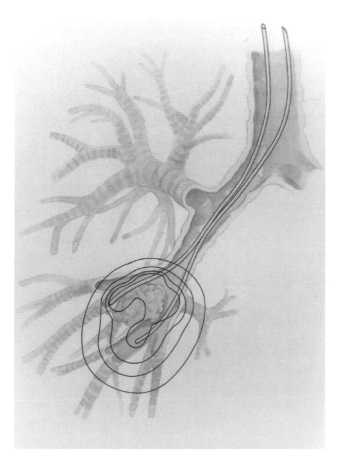

Figure 5.5 HDR endobronchial brachytherapy — note how the use of two catheters and dose optimization allows for precise irradiation of an irregular target volume. (Reproduced with the kind permission of Nucletron, Inc.)

Why we like the microSelectron HDR

- The small source size allows the source to negotiate a curve with a radius ≥ 1.5 cm.
- Maximum source extension of 1500 mm is available
- 300 points available for dose optimization; this allows the dose distribution to be tailored very precisely in relation to the target volume.
- Dwell times in increments of 0.1 s also improve the ability for dose optimization.
- Excellent after-sales service and support.

Tips and tricks

- Try to select the largest applicator compatible with the local anatomy. Applicators that are at least 5 Fr in size are the best.
- The entire system of the applicator and the connecting cable (which connects the applicator to the machine) should lie in a smooth curve. The source itself can negotiate a right angle, or even more acute curves, but care should be taken to prevent any kinking of the applicator as it curves.
- Use only gas sterilization for the applicators. All other methods of sterilization have the potential for creating a build-up within the applicator, and also for contamination of the source itself.
- To minimize the possibility of errors, use magnetic cards to program the afterloader, instead of manual entry of dwell positions and dwell times. The modern versions employ an integrated planning system, wherein the treatment plan is directly transferred to the microprocessor that controls the HDR unit and the source movement.

Review of literature

The effectiveness of endovascular brachytherapy, using a high dose-rate remote afterloader, to prevent post-angioplasty restenosis has been consistently confirmed in the laboratory setting, and the technique is now being evaluated in clinical trials. The first indications of clinical utility came from a pilot study in Europe. Thus, Schopohl et al reported on 28 patients with femoropopliteal restenosis, treated with angioplasty, stenting and post-PTA endovascular high dose-rate brachytherapy. At a follow-up period ranging up to 6 years, 21 of the 25 patients who were available for follow-up showed no evidence of restenosis. Similar results have also been reported from Vienna. Thus, in their pilot study of 10 patients with long segment femoropopliteal restenosis (mean length 16 cm, range 9–22 cm), Pokrajac et al delivered post-angioplasty endovascular radiation employing this HDR remote afterloader. A dose of 12 Gy was targeted to the inner intima. No stents were employed. A 12-month follow-up revealed a 60% patency rate in this population with a very unfavorable prognostic outlook. This was followed by a randomized study of angioplasty vs angioplasty plus endovascular radiation in patients with recurrent stenoses or any patient with lesion length > 5 cm. In all, 113 patients were enrolled and a dose of 12 Gy was prescribed to the vessel surface. No centering was employed. Mean lesion length treated was 15.7 cm. Follow up was mainly clinical with color duplex sonography, although about 60% of the patients also had a follow-up angiogram. Preliminary results show a recurrence rate of 49% in the control group vs 24% in the radiated arm. This has now evolved into an Austrian multi-center, randomized study with a design similar to the PARIS Trial (vide infra). The Swiss group (Greiner et al) is also conducting similar studies—an initial Phase I study consisted of patients receiving 12 Gy prescribed at a radial distance of 3 mm from the source. A second phase was started in parallel, as a randomized study of PTA with or without endovascular radiation, with the dose now being prescribed at a distance of 5 mm. The third phase is a four-arm study comparing PTA + aspirin, PTA + probucol, PTA + aspirin + probucol and PTA + aspirin + probucol + endovascular radiation. A total of 320 patients will be enrolled, and 14 Gy will be prescribed at the reference radius +2 mm. No stents or centering devices will be used.

This concept is currently undergoing validation in a number of trials in the USA. The Emory Clinic reported a pilot study on patients undergoing post-PTA endovascular high dose-rate brachytherapy in the femoropopliteal arteries and in the setting of compromised dialysis accesses. Their results seemed to confirm the German study. This work is being more rigorously validated by Waksman et al. Thus, the PARIS Trial is planned to study the clinical efficacy of remote afterloading high dose-rate endovascular brachytherapy in preventing post-angioplasty restenosis in the femoropopliteal arteries. The double-blinded, randomized design of this trial (described elsewhere in greater detail) will allow the objective assessment of the contribution of radiotherapy in improving the durability of the angioplasty in this setting. The group at the Scripps Clinic is also evaluating the feasibility and safety of this approach in a Phase I study of TIPS (transjugular intrahepatic portosystemic shunts)—15 patients will be enrolled and 10–30 Gy will be prescribed based on IVUS measurements.

Studies

Past	• Non-randomized study of post-PTA endovascular irradiation in femoropopliteal restenosis (Frankfurt, Germany) • Non-randomized study of post-PTA endovascular irradiation for femoropopliteal restenosis and for patients with compromised dialysis accesses (Emory Clinic, Atlanta, GA, USA)
Present/ Completed	• Phase I component of the PARIS Trial of high dose-rate endovascular brachytherapy following successful angioplasty in the femoropopliteal arteries (USA) • Vienna 01 Trial: Phase I study of high dose-rate endovascular brachytherapy following successful angioplasty in long segment, restenotic femoropopliteal lesions • Vienna 02 Trial: randomized study of angioplasty with or without endovascular brachytherapy in 113 patients with de novo (> 5 cm) and restenotic femoropopliteal lesions
Present/ Ongoing	• Multi-center, Austrian Trial: randomized study using the PARIS catheter, but including longer total occlusions, and employing a dose of 18 Gy to a distance = reference radius + 2 mm • PARIS Trial: a multi-institutional, randomized study of 300 patients with femoropopliteal stenoses. A special centering catheter is employed and a dose of 14 Gy is prescribed to a distance = reference radius + 2 mm • Swiss Trials: three-phase study in femoropopliteal stenoses, with a feasibility phase, a concurrent randomized study and a subsequent four-arm study randomizing patients to post-PTA aspirin, probucol, aspirin + probucol, or aspirin + probucol + radiation • Scripps TIPS Trial: Phase I study of post-PTA endovascular radiation in TIPS shunts, employing IVUS-based dose prescription

6. THE IR-192 RADIOACTIVE SEED RIBBON

Scripps Clinic and Research Foundation, La Jolla, CA, USA

Shirish K Jani, Vincent Massullo, Prabhakar Tripuraneni and Paul Teirstein

Description	Nylon ribbon containing an array of small, cylindrically shaped iridium-192 radioactive sources. Figure 6.1 shows a photograph of a typical Ir-192 seed ribbon for coronary brachytherapy application.

History	• **1981**	Best Medical International began production and supply of radioactive Ir-192 seeds embedded in nylon ribbons for the treatment of cancer
	• **Early 1995**	The Scripps Clinic initiated the first randomized clinical trial to evaluate the role of this device in treating coronary restenosis

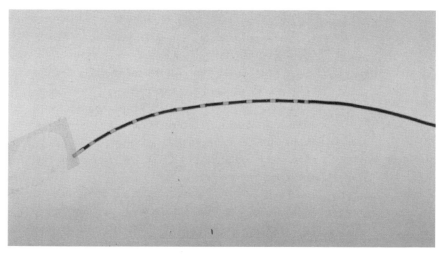

Figure 6.1 *Photograph of a Ir-192 source ribbon manufactured by Best Medical International.*

Technical specifications

Source composition	30% iridium 70% platinum
Source encapsulation	Stainless steel (0.02 cm)
Source dimension	Cylindrical; 0.05-cm diameter, 0.3-cm length
Source configuration	See Figure 6.2 for schematic drawing
Available from	In the USA: these sources are only available when embedded in nylon ribbon
Spacing between sources	Variable (typically 0–1 cm)
Available active length	Variable (typically 2–10 cm)
Available overall length	Variable (typically 100–300 cm)
Available activity	0.1–30 mCi per seed source
Iridium radioisotope	atomic number: 77 atomic mass: 192 emitted radiation: gamma energy range: 0.136–1.06 MeV (primarily 0.3–0.6 MeV) average gamma energy: 0.37 MeV half life: 74.2 days half value layers: ≈3 mm lead

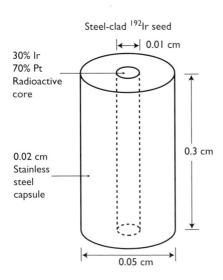

Figure 6.2 *Schematic drawing of an individual Ir-192 seed source.*

Tips and tricks

The Ir-192 seed sources are arranged in the nylon ribbon as shown in Figure 6.3. There is a 0.1-cm gap kept between the seeds which makes the active end of the ribbon flexible enough to negotiate it through tortuous paths when approaching coronary arteries. A guidewire embedded in the rest of the 300-cm long ribbon helps to push the active ribbon to its target through a catheter. The available source strength is high enough to limit the treatment time to < 20 min.

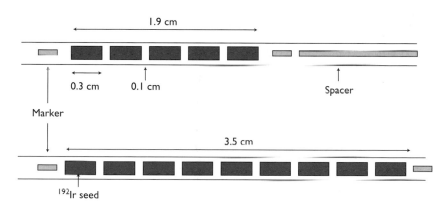

Figure 6.3 *Schematic drawing (not to scale) of an Ir-192 seed arrangement in nylon ribbon. These lengths of radioactive segment were initially chosen to match the required length of tissues to be irradiated around one or two Palmaz–Schatz stents.*

Indications for clinical use

At present, the Ir-192 ribbon manufactured by Best Medical International (Springfield, VA, USA) and available through Cordis Corporation (Warren, NJ, USA) is approved for investigational purposes, i.e. performing endovascular brachytherapy to prevent or reduce restenosis. A typical brachytherapy irradiation would be 15–25 min in duration for treating coronary restenosis. Figure 6.4 illustrates the clinical use of Ir-192 ribbon during the investigational phase of the Scripps I Trial on restenotic lesions.

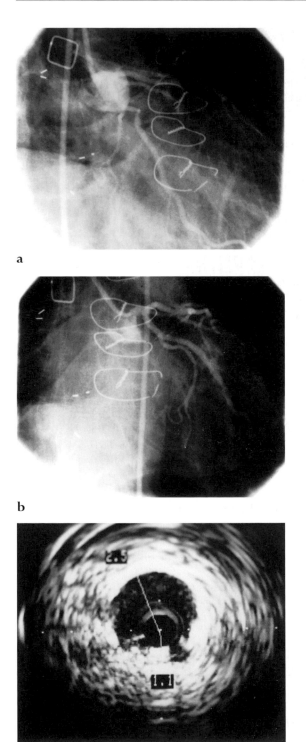

a

b

c

Figure 6.4 *A 55-year-old man with recurrent angina after percutaneous transluminal coronary angioplasty of the native coronary artery. (a) Restenosis in the left circumflex artery. (b) Angiogram after redilation and restenting using two Palmaz–Schatz stents. (c) Intravascular ultrasound image of the restented artery to obtain cross-sectional dimensions for radiotherapy dose prescription. (d) A cinefluorographic image during coronary irradiation showing a nine-seed Ir-192 ribbon spanning the stented region. (e) Six-month follow-up angiogram showing the irradiated segment of the left circumflex artery.*

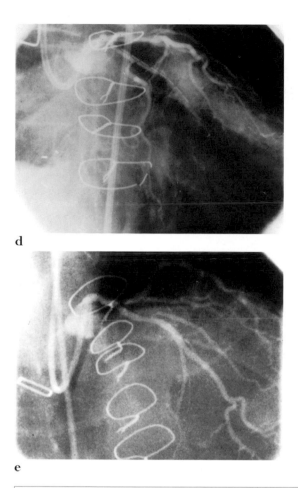

d

e

Why we like the Best Ir-192 seed ribbon

Gamma-radiation from an Ir-192 source provides a dose homogeneity
better than that of any beta source. Moreover, the presence of metallic
stent or calcification within arterial wall does not alter the dose
distribution around Ir-192 ribbon significantly.

Precautions

- When high activity of Ir-192 is employed to shorten the treatment
  time, it produces significant radiation exposure levels around the
  patient and the room. Portable radiation shields are used to provide
  proper radiation safety to staff.
- At present, the non-centered configuration of the Ir-192 ribbon
  delivers an uneven dose to the arterial wall around it.

Studies

Scripps I Trial (1995)
- 55 patients with known restenosis in coronary artery
- Randomized double-blinded study at Scripps Clinic, La Jolla, CA, USA
- Significant reduction in restenosis rate in the radiation arm

Scripps II Trial (1996–98)
- 105 patients with known restenosis in coronary artery
- Randomized double-blinded study at Scripps Clinic, La Jolla, CA, USA
- Completed enrollment—final results in 1999

Wrist Trial (1997)
- 130 patients with known restenosis in coronary artery
- Randomized double-blinded study at Washington Hospital, Washington, DC, USA
- Significant reduction in restenosis rate in the radiation arm

Gamma I Trial (1998)
- 252 patients with known restenosis in coronary artery
- Randomized double-blinded study
- Multi-center within the USA (Cordis Corp)
- Significant reduction in restenosis rate in the radiation arm

Gamma II Registry (1998)
- 125 patients with known restenosis in coronary artery
- Patient Registry—multi-center within the USA (Cordis Corp)
- Outcome pending

High risk patients Registry (1999)
- 60 patients with known restenosis in coronary artery
- Patient Registry—multi-center within the USA (Cordis Corp)
- Outcome pending

Scripps III Trial (1999)
- 250 patients with known restenosis in coronary artery
- To reduce stent thrombosis following Ir-192 brachytherapy
- Scripps Clinic, La Jolla, CA, USA
- Enrollment began in 1999

7. THE ANGIORAD™ SYSTEM

Vascular Therapies, United States Surgical Corporation, Norwalk, CT, USA

David Faxon and Sam Liprie

Definition	The Angiorad™ System has three components. A small and flexible source wire, a delivery catheter, and a manual delivery device which stores, advances and retracts the source wire (Figures 11.1 and 11.2).

History	• A unique flexible 0.014 inch iridium-192 source wire, developed by Sam Liprie in 1995 and tested in initial studies in Venezuela. • The delivery catheter and manual delivery device was developed by Vascular Therapies (Figure 11.3).

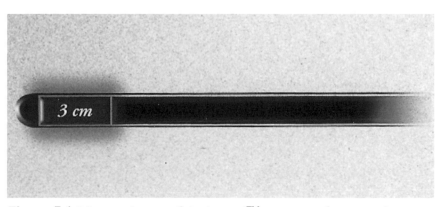

Figure 7.1 *Schematic drawing of the Angiorad™ source wire, featuring a 3 cm iridium-192 core inserted into the distal cavity of a .014 inch nitinol wire.*

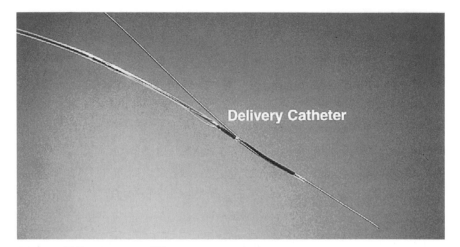

Figure 7.2 *The Angiorad™ delivery catheter, featuring a distal monorail section for the PTCA wire with a balloon lumen and a closed end lumen for the source wire. The catheter is compatible with 6 French guide catheters and features a .030 inch profile on a 3.2 French shaft.*

Indications for use

The unit is currently under the final phase of development. Please refer to package instructions for use.

Why I like my device

- The Angiorad™ System is simple yet eloquent
- The catheter performs similar to high performance PTCA balloon systems.
- It is able to reach distal coronary anatomy even in severe tortuosity and in small vessels and provides perfusion during treatment.
- The delivery catheter takes advantage of the source wire's high trackability and small size.
- The afterloader is small, compact and easy to use with safety features that allow rapid retrieval if necessary.

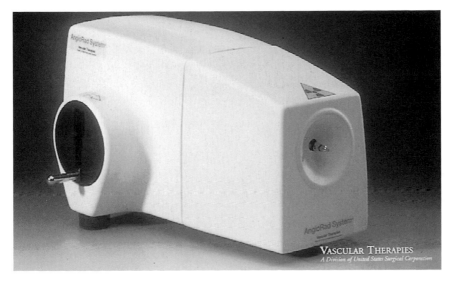

a

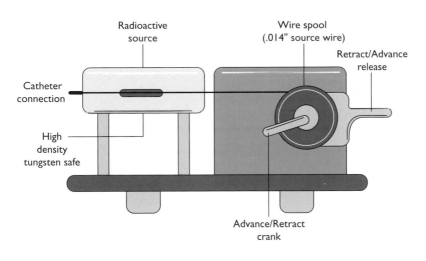

b

Figure 7.3 (a) and (b) show an illustration and schematic drawing of the the Angiorad™ manual delivery device which stores the source wire with its radioactive core. It features a manual crank for advancement and retraction of the source wire and a tungsten drum to shield the radioactive core. The unit has an automatic stopping mechanism and multiple safety locks for source replacement and unit service.

Key features

- Compatible with 6 French guide catheter
- Highly trackable catheter and source wire
- Simple to use manual delivery device
- Low exposure levels during delivery for a non-automated delivery device.

Planned indications for clinical use

The Angiorad™ System is designed to allow for multiple utility in delivering radiation to a site for the reduction of restenosis. Initial clinical trials will focus on small vessel disease and in-stent restenosis. Clinical trials are planned for the United States and Europe.

8. THE NUCLETRON PERIPHERAL VASCULAR BRACHYTHERAPY SYSTEM

Interventional Technologies, San Diego, CA, USA

Ron Waksman

Definition   This high dose-rate remote afterloader system (microSelectron HDR) delivers radiation (flexible, short, thin 192-Ir source) via an end lumen sheath placed in a centering segmented balloon catheter to the treated vessel site for prevention of restenosis.

History   Brasfield and Henschke reported the use of vascular brachytherapy as early as 1958 for irradiation of the parasternal mammary lymph nodes in the treatment of breast cancer.[1] Remote afterloading brachytherapy has been in use for cancer treatment since 1975. Restenosis is the major limitation of percutaneous transcatheter angioplasty (PTA) of narrowed vessels.[2] Endovascular radiation was shown to reduce the restenosis rate both in animal models and human feasibility trials. The pioneering work of using endovascular radiation for prevention of restenosis in the peripheral vascular system was initiated in 1991 by Schopohl and Leirmann. They treated patients following PTA of narrowed stented arteries using the microSelectron-HDR afterloader. Based on their studies it was suggested that vascular brachytherapy for this application was safe and probably efficacious.[3] The encouraging results of this study led other investigators to conduct feasibility trials in the peripheral vascular system[4] and to develop a centering delivery catheter system to provide a uniform dose to the vessel wall. This centering catheter is currently in use in a multi-center study protocol entitled PARIS (Peripheral Artery Radiation Investigational Study) which was approved by the FDA and began in 1997.

Advantages of the remote afterloading system for vascular brachytherapy

- The remote afterloading system drives the radiation source quickly to the treatment site, avoiding radiation exposure of non-treated arteries.
- Radiation exposure to clinical personnel is eliminated by remotely programming the automatic advancement of the radiation source to the treatment site from a shielded safe.
- The radiation dose can be controlled and shaped using the computerized afterloader device to accurately adjust the source position and treatment time.
- The afterloader continually monitors the radiation dose and automatically retracts the source into the shielded safe after completion of treatment.
- The treatment time is automatically adapted for the radioactive decay of the source.
- The afterloader can handle a very high activity source (10 Ci), which results in a short treatment time.

The PARIS centering catheter system (Figures 8.1 and 8.2)

The peripheral brachytherapy centering catheter is manufactured by Guidant Corporation (Santa Clara, CA, USA) and is a double-lumen catheter with multiple centering balloons near its distal tip. One lumen is for inflation of the centering balloons, the second lumen is for the guide wire and for the closed end lumen sheath which is introduced following removal of the guide wire once the catheter is in position. The inflated balloons engage the walls of the vessels to allow centering. The shaft diameter is 7 Fr and the balloons are 4–8 mm in diameter and 10–20 cm in length.

The source, the dose and the dosimetry

The source used for peripheral arteries is gamma ^{192}Ir that can penetrate vessels with a larger diameter. The source is short (3.5 mm length and 0.6 mm thin), mounted on an ultra-flexible cable and is certified to 25 000 transfers.

- The dose in the PARIS protocol is 14 Gy.
- The target depth +1/2 of the reference diameter +2 mm.
- The target length + lesion length + safety margin of 10 mm.

- Step size = 5 mm.
- Active length + target length + distal and proximal 5-mm margin.

Clinical studies (Table 8.1)

The Frankfurt experience
This was the first pilot study of endovascular radiation, which was conducted in 30 patients with in-stent restenosis in their superficial femoral arteries

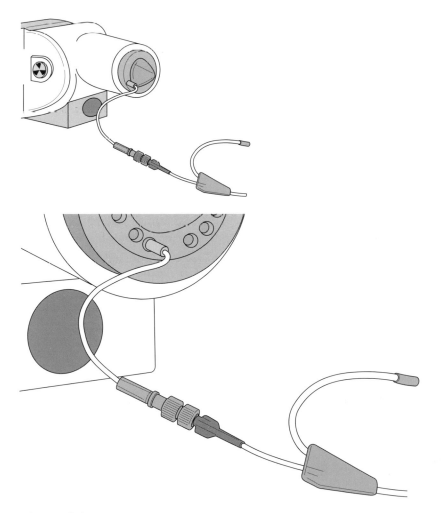

Figure 8.1 *The Nucletron microSelectron-HDR PARIS brachytherapy centering catheter system.*

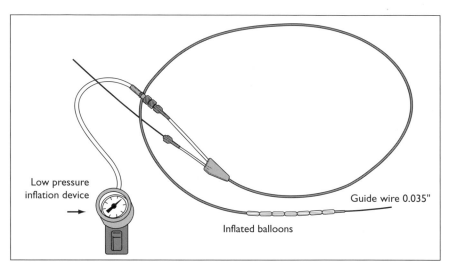

a

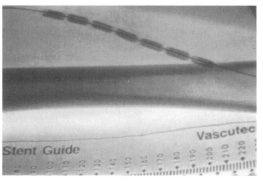

b

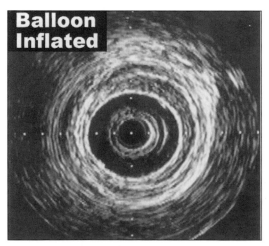

c

Figure 8.2 The centering catheter: (a) overall system; (b) angiographic image of the inflated centering catheter in the SFA; (c) intravascular ultrasound image of the inflated balloon in the SFA.

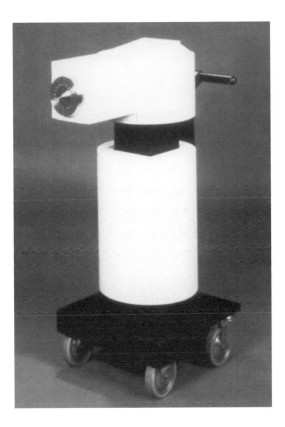

Figure 8.3
The microSelectron-HDR afterloader.

(SFA).[3] The patients underwent atherectomy and PTA followed by endovascular radiation using the microSelectron-HDR and a non-centering catheter. The source was ^{192}Ir and the dose was 12 Gy prescribed to 3 mm distance, while the actual dose varied from 8 to 28 Gy. There were no reported adverse effects from the radiation treatment up to 7 years follow-up. The 5-year patency rate of the target vessel was 82% with 3/28 (11%) stenosis within the treated segment. Late total occlusion developed in 2/28 patients (7%) after 16 and 37 months respectively.[4]

The Vienna experience

The effectiveness of the Nucletron microSelectron-HDR system was tested in a randomized placebo-controlled trial in Vienna using ^{192}Ir, a non-centering closed end lumen catheter and a prescribed dose of 12 Gy in 100 patients following PTA to the SFA and the popliteal arteries. This study demonstrated a 50% reduction in the clinical restenosis rate in the irradiated group versus controls.[5]

Table 8.1 Peripheral studies using the nucletron microSelectron-HDR

Treated vessel	Reference/ Study	Delivery catheter	Radiation source	Dose (Gy)	Results and status
Superficial femoral artery (SFA)	3,4	Non-centered 5.0 Fr catheter	192-Ir	12	25 patients completed 5 years follow-up with 82% patency at the treatment site
AV dialysis shunts	7	Non-centered 5.0 Fr catheter	192-Ir	14	11 patients, 18 lesions, with 40% patency rate at 44 weeks
SFA	5 randomized placebo-control	Non-centered 5.0 Fr catheter, closed-end lumen	192-Ir	12	50% angiographic reduction in the restenosis rate at 6 months in the irradiated group
SFA	6 PARIS feasibility	Centering 7.0 Fr segmented balloon catheter	192-Ir	14	12% clinical and angiographic restenosis at 12 months
SFA	PARIS randomized placebo-control	Centering 7.0 Fr segmented balloon catheter	192-Ir	14	300 patients will complete enroll-ment in 2000

The PARIS Trial

PARIS is the first FDA-approved double-blind randomized trial with and without intravascular radiation in the peripheral system. This study will investigate 300 patients undergoing PTA to SFA lesions between 5 and 15 cm in length. In the feasibility phase of the PARIS Trial all patients were treated with radiation following PTA. After the intervention the PARIS centering catheter was introduced and positioned to cover the angioplasty site. The actual radiation treatment is performed in the radiation oncology suite using the microSelectron-HDR afterloader. The isotope used for the study was [192]Ir (maximum of 10 Ci in activity), and the prescribed dose was 14 Gy to a depth of 2 mm into the vessel wall. Forty patients were enrolled in the feasibility study. Lesions at the SFA measuring 5–15 cm underwent successful PTA. The position of the centering device was verified to be stable after patient transport to the radiation suite, and the radiation therapy was successfully delivered to 35/40 patients. The 6-month angiographic follow-up was completed for 30 patients and a restenosis rate of 13.3% clinical restenosis at 1 year was reported in 12% of patients.[6] The randomization phase for this study is scheduled to be completed by the end of 2000 and results are expected in 2001. The outcome of this study will determine the future of endovascular radiation therapy for prevention of restenosis in the peripheral vascular system.

Feasibility studies for arteriovenous dialysis shunts

Waksman et al conducted a feasibility study in 11 patients with recurrent narrowing of the arteriovenous (AV) dialysis graft.[7] Following PTA the microSelectron-HDR was used to deliver the radiation via a non-centering end lumen 5-Fr catheter. All procedures were successful, with no procedural or in-hospital complications. However, the patency rate at the treated site at 44 weeks was only 40%. This was explained by late thrombosis and may be caused by the lack of a centering system in this study.

Potential application for the Nucletron system

- Femoral arteries de novo
- Femoral arteries in-stent restenosis
- Renal arteries
- Transjugular intrahepatic porto-systemic shunting (TIPS) procedures
- AV dialysis shunt stenosis
- Subclavian vein stenosis

References

1. Brasfield RD, Henscke UK. Treatment of internal mammary lymph nodes by implantation of radioisotopes into internal mammary artery. *Radiology* 1958; **70**:259.

2. Hunink MFM, Magruder CD, Meyerovitz MF et al. Risks and benefits of femoro-popliteal percutaneous balloon angioplasty. *J Vasc Surg* 1993; **17**:183–194.

3. Liermann DD, Boettcher HD, Kollatch J et al. Prophylactic endovascular radiotherapy to prevent intimal hyperplasia after stent implantation in femoro-popliteal arteries. *Cardiovasc Intervent Radiol* 1994; **17**:12–16.

4. Schoppel D, Liermann LJ, Pohlit R et al. 192-Ir endovascular brachytherapy for avoidance of intimal hyperplasia after percutaneous transluminal angioplasty and stent implantation in peripheral vessels: years of experience. *Int J Radiat Oncol Biol Phys* 1996; **36**:835–840.

5. Minar E. SFA brachytherapy: The Vienna experience. *Cardiovascular Radiation Therapy III, Syllabus* 1999: 431 (abstract).

6. Waksman R, Laird JR, Benenati J et al. Intravascular radiation for prevention of restenosis after angioplasty of narrowed femoral-popliteal arteries: Preliminary six month results of a feasibility study. *Circulation* 1998; **98**:17,I-66:331 (abstract).

7. Waksman R, Crocker IA, Kikeri D, Lumsden A, MacDonald JM, Martin LG. Long term results of endovascular radiation therapy for prevention of restenosis in the peripheral vascular system. *Circulation* 1996; **94**:8,I-300:1745 (abstract).

9. THE BETA-CATH™ SYSTEM

Novoste Corporation, Norcross, GA, USA

Raoul Bonan, Richard diMonda and Richard A Hillstead

Description

The Beta-Cath™ system is a proprietary catheter-based delivery system that delivers localized beta-radiation to a coronary artery at the site of coronary intervention. The system is composed of two separate components (Figure 9.1).

- The *transfer device* containing a radiation source train: a multiple-use, hand-held instrument designed to shield, store, and transport the radiation source train. The transfer device uses sterile water to hydraulically deliver the sources within the delivery catheter to the treatment site. The radiation

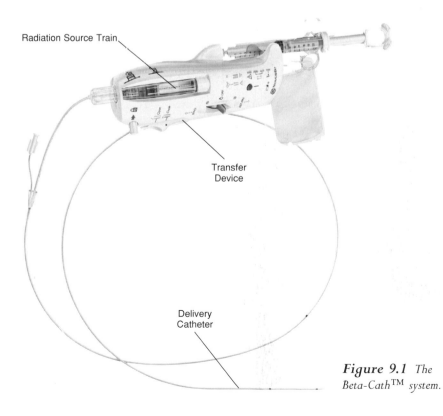

Radiation Source Train

Transfer Device

Delivery Catheter

Figure 9.1 *The Beta-Cath™ system.*

source train is comprised of several miniature cylindrical sealed sources containing Sr-90/Y-90, which are pure beta emitters.

• The *delivery catheter*: a single-use, multi-lumen catheter (over-the-wire or rapid exchange design) that is positioned at the coronary artery treatment site and allows the radiation source train to be delivered and returned to the transfer device.

The Beta-Cath™ system is used in a cardiac catheterization laboratory immediately after percutaneous transluminal coronary angioplasty (PTCA). After removing the angioplasty catheter, the interventional cardiologist uses the existing guidewire and guiding catheter to direct the delivery catheter into the coronary anatomy of the patient until the radiopaque marker bands of the catheter are positioned at the balloon injury site. With the use of sterile water, the radiation source train is then hydraulically delivered from the transfer device to the treatment site in about 3 s through the source train lumen of the delivery catheter. The radiation sources remain at the treatment site for approximately 3–4 min to deliver a predetermined dose of β-radiation to the target tissue. The radiation sources are then returned to the transfer device by applying positive hydraulic pressure through the delivery catheter's fluid return lumen. The Beta-Cath™ system functions as a closed loop system; i.e. delivery fluid is not injected into the patient's coronary arteries and the radiation source train does not come in contact with the patient's blood or tissue (Figure 9.2).

Upon completion of the procedure, the single-use delivery catheter is disposed of according to hospital policy. The radiation source train is housed within the transfer device and stored in a designated radiation storage site until the next procedure.

The Novoste Beta-Cath™ system is the first vascular brachytherapy product to receive a CE mark in Europe and is commercially available in select European and Middle Eastern markets, Australia, and New Zealand.

Future additions to the Beta-Cath™ system product family currently under development include products designed for small vessel, diffuse disease and peripheral vascular applications.

History
- **1994** Novoste's first prototype of the Beta-Cath™ system design was employed in preclinical studies at Emory University Hospital. The device was used in domestic pigs following balloon overstretch injury, with doses ranging from 7 to 56 Gy. A dose-dependent reduction of neointimal formation was observed.
- **1995** Additional preclinical studies of the Beta-Cath™ system in the swine model in conjunction with coronary artery stenting also demonstrated marked inhibition of neointimal formation.
- **January 1996** The US feasibility clinical trial, the Beta Energy Restenosis Trial (BERT-1), was initiated at Emory University Hospital. The trial was later expanded to include the Rhode Island Hospital.
- **February 1997** The international clinical trial, the BERT-1.5 study, was initiated at the Montreal Heart Institute in Canada, followed shortly afterwards by the Thoraxcenter at Erasmus University in Rotterdam, The Netherlands.
- **March 1997** Spencer B King III, MD presented very encouraging preliminary results from the BERT-1 study at the *46th Annual Scientific Session of the American College of Cardiology* meeting in Anaheim, CA, USA.
- **July 1997** Novoste initiated a prospective, randomized, placebo-controlled, multicenter clinical trial, the Beta-Cath™ System Trial. This study is investigating the role of beta-radiation in the prevention of restenosis in de novo PTCA and provisional stent patients.
- **July 1998** Novoste initiated a registry clinical trial, the Beta Radiation In Europe (BRIE) Trial. This study is investigating the use of beta-radiation in single and multi-vessel disease patients.
- **August 1998** Novoste received CE mark approval to market the Beta-Cath™ system in Europe, establishing the Beta-Cath™ system as the first commercially available vascular brachytherapy device in the world.
- **September 1998** Novoste initiated a prospective, randomized, placebo-controlled, multi-center clinical trial, the STents And Radiation Therapy (START) Trial. This study is investigating the role of beta-radiation in the treatment of in-stent restenosis; the patient enrollment phase was completed in April 1999.
- **June 1999** Novoste initiated a prospective, non-randomized, retrospective placebo-controlled, multi-center clinical trial, the START 40 Trial. This study is investigating the use of the 40-mm radiation source train in treating in-stent restenosis patients with an expected 10-mm margin of radiation on each end of the injury length.

Technical specifications

Delivery catheter

Usable life	Single life
Outer diameter	5 French
Wire requirements	0.014 in coronary guidewire
Catheter length	Standard: 135 cm working length, 155 cm overall
	XL: 135 cm working length, 275 cm overall
Lumens	Three lumen designs: two closed lumens (radiation source train lumen and fluid return lumen) and one open lumen (guidewire lumen)

Radiation source train

Radioactive material	Sr-90/Y-90
Half-life	28 years
Usable life	Multiple-use; 250 uses per train prior to routine maintenance
Prescription point	2 mm from the center-line of the axis of the train
Prescription dose	14–20 Gy (based on the size of the vessel and if stent is in place)
Radiation type	Beta-radiation
Train components	Independent cylindrical sealed sources with one inactive gold marker seed at each end
Train length	30 mm, 40 mm (additional train lengths anticipated)

Transfer device

Size	Hand-held unit
Safety features	Electronic sensing of radiation source train location, source gate interlock, catheter disconnect interlock
Shielding	100% shielding of beta-radiation
Usable life	Multiple-use
Isotope delivery	Manual hydraulic control with attached sterile water-filled syringe

Features and benefits of the Beta-Cath™ system

The Beta-Cath™ system was originally and specifically designed to treat coronary restenosis with intracoronary β-radiation in the cardiac catheterization laboratory setting. Because of this design approach, the device has many features that are attractive to both interventional cardiologists and radiation therapists, as listed below.

• Beta-radiation—Because β-radiation can be effectively absorbed by man-made materials, it is easily shielded within the transfer device. Additionally, no catheterization laboratory radiation shielding modifications are required. Furthermore, the depth of penetration of the β-radiation is closely aligned with the geometry of the coronary artery, greatly minimizing the exposure of adjacent tissues.

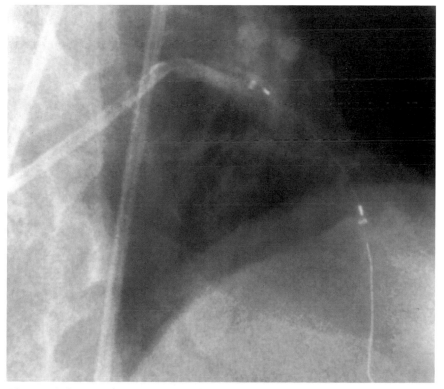

Figure 9.2 *Angiogram of Beta-Cath™ delivery catheter and radiation source train in coronary artery.*

- Designed for safety—Because the Beta-Cath™ system uses β-radiation, radiation exposure to healthcare workers and patients is minimal. In fact, the total body exposure received by the patient during one procedure is < 1/100 of the exposure received during routine fluoroscopy. In addition, the physician may remain at the patient's bedside throughout the procedure. The device also has several built-in safety features such as:
  - proprietary connector mechanism on the delivery catheter which must be properly attached to the transfer device in order for the radiation source train to exit the transfer device
  - sensors to detect the position of the radiation source train in the transfer device
  - interlock mechanisms to protect against inadvertent catheter disconnection
  - the system is manually operated, so that the physician maintains complete control over catheter placement and isotope movement.
- Variable length radiation source train—The radiation source train is available in a variety of lengths. This feature provides the clinician with the appropriate radiation treatment length to cover the vessel injury area with sufficient margin and effectively deliver the radiation to the treatment site.
- Long half-life isotope—Inventory planning is simplified because the isotope is reusable and has a long shelf-life. Additionally, dosing calculations are very straightforward because the activity of the isotope remains essentially constant for months.
- Passive centering delivery catheter—The 5-Fr delivery catheter is designed to be appropriately sized to the coronary artery minimum lumen diameter (MLD) in order to provide homogeneous dose delivery to the target tissue while, at the same time, allowing distal perfusion around the delivery catheter during the radiation treatment.
- Short treatment times—The recommended radiation dose can be delivered by the Beta-Cath™ system in approximately 3–5 min, thereby minimizing the risk of ischemia that may occur with occlusive, long dwell time systems.
- Cost-effectiveness—The radiation source train can be reused many times owing to the long half-life of the isotope and because the radiation source train never comes in contact with patient's blood. As a result, procedure costs are reduced. Also, catheterization laboratory throughput should not be adversely impacted owing to the short treatment times required by the Beta-Cath™ system.

Summary of clinical trials

Novoste initiated an FDA-approved feasibility clinical trial, the BERT-1 study, in the USA in January 1996. Patients with single vessel, de novo lesions were enrolled into the trial, the purpose of which was to evaluate the safety and clinical feasibility of the Beta-Cath™ system at three radiation doses: 12, 14, and 16 Gy. The trial was designed to treat a patient population similar to the Lovastatin Restenosis Trial, so that historical control data would be available for comparison. Each of the treated BERT patients received balloon angioplasty before receiving vascular brachytherapy, and then underwent a follow-up angiogram within 6 months of the initial treatment.

Novoste expanded its feasibility clinical trial outside the USA in February 1997 with the BERT-1.5 study. This trial used the same protocol as the BERT-1 study and included two additional clinical sites.

Of the 85 patients enrolled in the BERT study, 82 successfully received vascular brachytherapy with the Beta-Cath™ system. Of these, 78 returned for angiographic follow-up 6 months after the procedure and exhibited a restenosis rate at the lesion site of 17%. This represents a >50% improvement in restenosis rate when compared with the historical control group, which did not received vascular brachytherapy. Additionally, the data demonstrated a >75% improvement in the 'late loss index,' a measure of how much of the artery enlargement achieved by angioplasty is lost within 6 months of the procedure. There were no major complications associated with the use of vascular brachytherapy in this study (Figure 9.3).

Another important finding occurred in a subgroup of 13 patients who received coronary stents as a 'bail-out' device to address acute complications, which can occur with angioplasty procedures. Within the bail-out stent subgroup, a restenosis rate of 8% was observed at the lesion site, which suggests a major improvement from restenosis rates typically observed in similar patients. Results for the entire study group, as evaluated by the independent angiographic core lab, are summarized in Table 9.1.

The largest clinical trial sponsored by Novoste Corporation is the Beta-Cath™ System Trial. This trial, which commenced in July 1997, is a prospective, randomized, placebo-controlled, triple-masked study to evaluate the safety and efficacy of the Beta-Cath™ system in native coronary arteries. The patient enrollment phase of this trial is expected to be complete in October 1999. The Beta-Cath™ System Trial was initially designed to include approximately 1100 patients. The trial has been extended to 1450 patients at over 60 medical centers worldwide to evaluate the effect of extended anti-platelet therapy in reducing late stent thrombosis associated with new stent placement. Patients who have undergone either elective PTCA or are

75

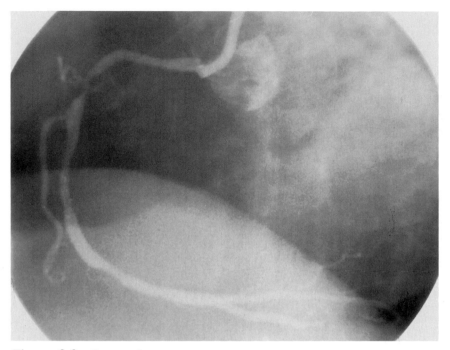

Figure 9.3a *Pre-procedure angiogram.*

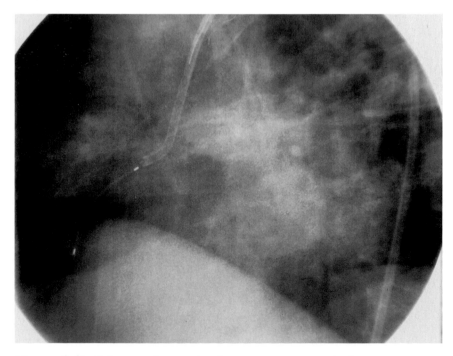

Figure 9.3b *Delivery catheter with radiation source train at the lesion.*

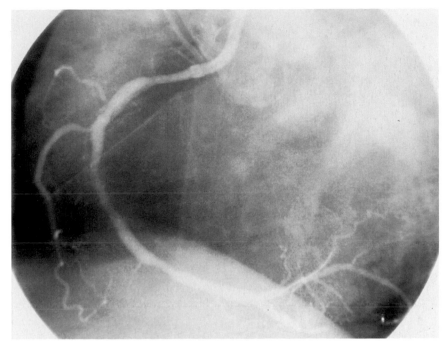

Figure 9.3c Post-radiation angiogram.

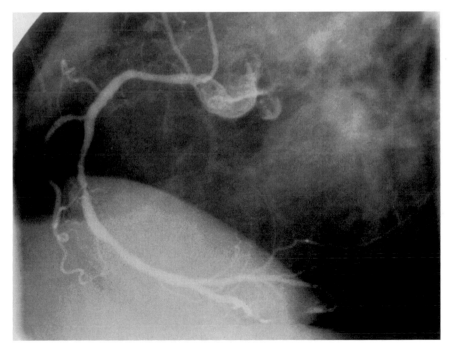

Figure 9.3d Six-month angiogram.

Table 9.1 Beta Energy Restenosis Trial (BERT) results.

Parameter	BERT (all doses)	BERT (14 and 16 Gy)	Lovastatin control group
Number of patients	78	52	161
Restenosis at lesion site (% of patients)	17%	15%	42%
Late loss index	9%	4%	43%
Number of patients receiving stents	13	9	0*
Stent restenosis at lesion site (% of patients)	8%	0	NA

*Coronary stents were not commercially available at the time of the Lovastatin Restenosis Trial.

candidates for provisional stent placement are eligible for the study and these patients may have either de novo or restenotic lesions. Each patient receives an 8-month follow-up evaluation to determine overall clinical event rates and angiographic restenosis rates.

In September 1998, Novoste initiated the STents And Radiation Therapy (START) Trial. This prospective, randomized, placebo-controlled, triple-masked trial is designed to evaluate the safety and efficacy of the Beta-Cath™ system in the treatment of in-stent restenosis. The patient enrollment phase of this trial was completed in April 1999, with over 450 patients enrolled. The 8-month follow-up angiographic evaluation and data analysis are expected to be complete in early 2000.

Other Novoste-sponsored clinical trials worldwide include: Beta Radiation In Europe (BRIE), a registry trial investigating the use of the Beta-Cath™ system in multi-vessel disease; START 40, investigating the use of the 40-mm radiation source train in patients presenting with in-stent restenosis; and REgistry NOvoste (RENO), a post-market surveillance registry trial.

Review of published animal studies

Initial pre-clinical studies were performed with commercially available products, including an Ir-192 wire. Later, preclinical studies included use of the Beta-Cath™ system. The results of the preclinical studies were presented at various interventional cardiology symposia and published in the journal *Circulation*[1–3].

Table 9.2 Results of computer-assisted histomorphometric analysis of sections from arteries of pigs in control and radiation-treated groups[1]

Parameter	Control	3.5 Gy	7 Gy	7 Gy delayed for 2 days	14 Gy
Number of arteries	20	10	10	11	8
Maximal intimal thickness (mm)	0.47 ± 0.21	0.47 ± 0.09	0.37 ± 0.18	0.27 ± 0.10	0.22 ± 0.12
Intimal area (mm²)	0.96 ± 0.70	1.23 ± 0.47	0.77 ± 0.44	0.48 ± 0.25	0.33 ± 0.35
IA/FL ratio	0.59 ± 0.23	0.38 ± 0.21	0.42 ± 0.16	0.24 ± 0.10	0.17 ± 0.16

Study 1[1]

Normal domestic pigs underwent balloon overstretch injury of their coronary arteries to simulate the human restenosis response. A high-activity Ir-192 source, a gamma emitter, was introduced at the injury site and left in place for a time sufficient to deliver one of three doses: 3.5, 7 or 14 Gy. To test the impact of delayed treatment, a 7-Gy dose was given to a group of animals 2 days after the overstretch injury. Fourteen days after treatment, tissue sections were measured to determine neointimal formation and the amount of injury was normalized by the ratio of intimal area to medial fracture length (IA/FL). To test the late effect and safety of endovascular irradiation, 7 or 14 Gy were given in mini-swine coronary arteries after injury as well as in non-injured carotid arteries; this group was followed up for 6 months.

At follow-up, all arteries treated with radiation demonstrated significantly decreased neointima formation compared with control arteries. A dose–response relationship was demonstrated, and delay of treatment by 2 days appeared to augment the inhibitory effect. The durability of the effect was also exhibited in the treated group after 6 months of follow-up.

Study 2[1]

The objective of this experiment was to determine whether β-radiation would have similar inhibitory effects to those of γ-radiation in reducing neointima formation in the swine restenosis model. Normal domestic pigs underwent balloon overstretch injury in their coronary arteries, and a flexible system was

Table 9.3 Results of computer-assisted histomorphometric analysis of sections from arteries of pigs in control and radiation-treated groups[2]

Parameter	Control	7 Gy	14 Gy	28 Gy	56 Gy
Number of arteries	16	9	9	2	2
Maximal intimal thickness (mm)	0.47 ± 0.15	0.40 ± 0.18	0.34 ± 0.23	0.23 ± 0.14	0.08 ± 0.09
Luminal area (mm²)	1.91 ± 0.85	2.01 ± 0.82	2.46 ± 1.20	3.85 ± 0.77	3.70 ± 1.36
Intimal area (mm²)	1.09 ± 0.70	0.81 ± 0.49	0.58 ± 0.54	0.47 ± 0.55	0.10 ± 0.15
IA/FL ratio	0.47 ± 0.25	0.34 ± 0.18	0.19 ± 0.20	0.08 ± 0.09	0.02 ± 0.02

used to advance a train of encapsulated Sr-90/Y-90 sources to the distal end of the catheter, where it remained for a time sufficient to deliver doses ranging from 7 to 56 Gy at a prescription point depth of 2 mm. Fourteen days after treatment, tissue sections were measured to determine neointima formation, and the amount of injury was normalized by the IA/FL ratio.

The results of the two studies involving β- and γ-radiation were very similar. In the former study, there was a significant decrease in neointimal formation in arteries receiving β-radiation compared with the control arteries. The ratio IA/FL was inversely proportional to the delivered dose, demonstrating a dose–response relationship. However, no further inhibitory effect was seen above 28 Gy.

From a safety perspective, there was no evidence of significant necrosis or excessive fibrosis in the coronary arteries or adjacent myocardium. Furthermore, the total body exposure to the pig and exposure to the healthcare staff was dramatically lower than with previous experiments using γ-radiation.

Study 3[1]

The objective of this experiment was to determine whether endovascular irradiation would decrease neointima formation in porcine arteries that received coronary stents. A total of 12 pigs were treated with either Sr-90/Y-90, receiving a dose of 14 Gy. Tantalum stents were implanted into the irradiated vessels, as well as in control vessels, which received no radiation treatment.

At the 28-day follow-up, the luminal area was significantly increased and the neointimal area was significantly decreased in both radiation treatment groups compared with controls, demonstrating that endovascular radiation treatment is also compatible with stent placement in pig coronary arteries.

References

1. Walsman R, Robinson KA, Crocker IR et al. Endovascular low-dose irradiation inhibits neointima formation after coronary artery balloon injury in swine—a possible role for radiation therapy in restenosis prevention. *Circulation* 1995; **91**:1533–1539.

2. Waksman R, Robinson KA, Crocker IR et al. Intracoronary low-dose β-irradiation inhibits neointima formation after coronary artery balloon injury in the swine restenosis model. *Circulation* 1995; **92**:3025–3031.

3. Waksman R, Robinson KA, Crocker IR et al. Intracoronary radiation before stent implantation inhibits neointima formation in stented porcine coronary studies. *Circulation* 1995; **92**:1383–1386.

10. THE GUIDANT GALILEO™ INTRAVASCULAR RADIOTHERAPY SYSTEM

Guidant Corporation, Vascular Intervention, Houston, TX, USA

Albert E Raizner, Robert P Eno and Richard V Calfee

Description The Galileo™ intravascular radiotherapy system consists of three components:

- A source wire, containing ^{32}P, a pure beta-emitting isotope sealed in the distal tip (Figure 10.1).
- A source delivery unit (SDU), or afterloader, which stores and shields the source wire, calculates the dosimetry, and automatically advances and retracts the wire (Figure 10.2).
- A centering catheter, which contains a dedicated dead-end lumen through which the source wire travels. The centering catheter has a spiral balloon that centers the source wire within the artery and allows for perfusion during the procedure. The catheter is highly flexible and is designed to navigate tortuous anatomy (Figure 10.3).

Several changes to the Galileo™ system are in development, including:

- an automatic stepping source
- an expanded range of centering catheter diameters and lengths as well as alternative balloon designs
- modifications to allow the system to treat large diameter vessels, including superficial femoral arteries.

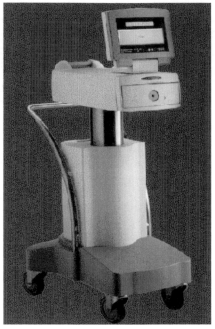

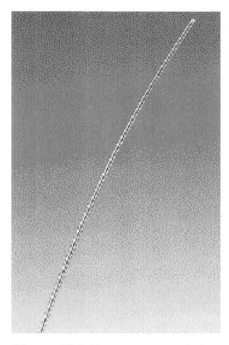

Figure 10.1 *The source wire with the beta emitter, ^{32}P, encapsulated in the distal 27 mm of this 0.018-inch Nitinol hypotube.*

Figure 10.2 *The source delivery unit (afterloader) calculates radiation treatment time and uses touch-screen technology to facilitate operator use. It provides for 'hands-off' delivery of radiotherapy.*

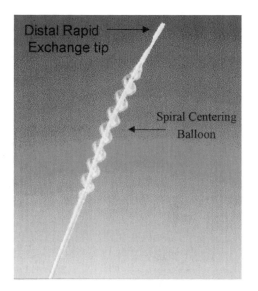

Distal Rapid Exchange tip

Spiral Centering Balloon

Figure 10.3 *The Guidant Galileo™ centering catheter showing the spiral balloon inflated. The distal rapid exchange tip incorporates a guidewire lumen for passage of the catheter over standard coronary guidewires.*

History	• 1992	Prototype catheter designed to provide passage of a radioactive source to an angioplasty site in a coronary artery.
	• 1993	Studies initiated in the porcine model of coronary restenosis at Baylor College of Medicine using ^{192}Ir. These studies established the efficacy of intracoronary radiotherapy in the inhibition of restenosis.
	• 1994	Centering catheter and a source wire using ^{32}P developed. Extensive animal investigations conducted using 3 mm and 27 mm active source lengths. These studies demonstrated that ^{32}P, a beta emitter, inhibited restenosis in balloon-injured (Figure 10.4) and stent-injured (Figure 10.5) porcine coronary arteries.
	• September 1997	US Food and Drug Administration (FDA) approval to initiate Phase I clinical trials in humans.
	• October 28, 1997	First human use of the Guidant intravascular radiotherapy system performed at Baylor College of Medicine and Methodist Hospital, Houston, TX, USA.
	• November 1997	The PREVENT trial, a randomized, placebo-controlled safety and feasibility study began.
	• May 1998	Enrollment in the PREVENT trial completed.
	• August 1998	First patient enrolled in INHIBIT, a pivotal trial investigating the ability of the Guidant intravascular radiotherapy system to reduce the rates of restenosis in patients with in-stent restenosis.
	• November 1999	The final results of the PREVENT trial presented at the American Heart Association Annual Scientific Session in Atlanta, GA, USA. A summary of these results is given below in 'Synopsis of clinical trials'.

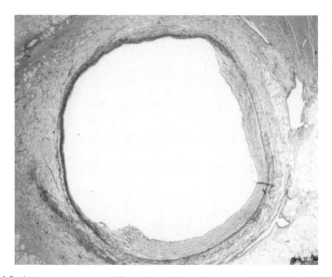

Figure 10.4 *Coronary artery of a swine subjected to extensive balloon injury and treated with intravascular brachytherapy with ^{32}P at a dose of 3500 cGy to the adventitia (equivalent to 2000 cGy to 1 mm into the artery wall). Note the absence of neointima, whose growth was inhibited by radiotherapy. There is thinning of the media at the point of maximal injury.*

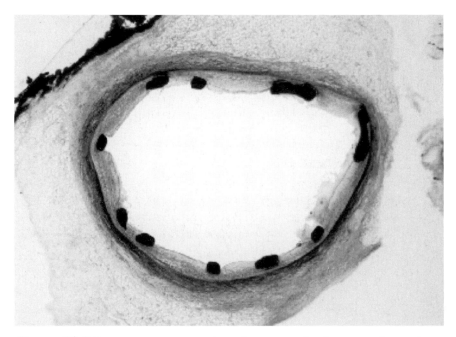

Figure 10.5 *Swine coronary artery subjected to stent-induced injury and treated with ^{32}P at a dose of 3500 cGy to the adventitia at the time of injury. There is minimal neointima formation and a widely patent lumen.*

Technical specifications

Source wire

Material	Nitinol
Diameter	0.018 inch
Source	^{32}P
Source configuration	Encapsulated
Source length	27 mm
Source activity	Up to 300 mCi

Centering catheter

Type	Distal rapid exchange
Configuration	Spiral (helical) balloon
Catheter length	135 cm
Balloon length (marker to marker)	27 mm
Shaft size	3.9 Fr
Balloon profile	< 3.9 Fr
Balloon inflation pressure	4 ± 1 atm
Balloon diameters (nominal)	2.5, 3.0, 3.5 mm

Source delivery unit

Mode of operation	Touch-screen control
Security controls	Password protection, key access
Method of dwell time calculation	Automatic, based on physician input of reference vessel diameter
Method of wire advancement	Automatically delivered by motor drive mechanism
Safety features	• Emergency back-up motor • Manual retract • No single-point radiation failure mechanism • Auto-retract with emergency stop button

Indications for use

The Guidant Galileo™ intravascular radiotherapy system is intended to deliver a controlled dose of radiation from a beta-emitting source safely and precisely to the target arterial segment immediately following an interventional procedure, with the intention of reducing the incidence of restenosis. At the time of writing, the Galileo™ system has not received regulatory approval and is not available for sale in any country. Guidant is pursuing a series of clinical trials to demonstrate the safety and efficacy of the Galileo™ intravascular radiotherapy system in a series of high-risk indications, starting with in-stent restenosis.

Tips and tricks

- Institutions considering the use of the Galileo™ intravascular radiotherapy system should ensure that a well-functioning team—including representatives from interventional cardiology, radiation oncology, and radiation safety—is in place.
- The Galileo™ intravascular radiotherapy system has been designed specifically for use in a cardiac catheterization laboratory, while drawing on proven afterloader technology used in radiation oncology. The system uses beta-radiation, a touch-screen control, and equipment familiar to interventional cardiology to ensure that the radiotherapy procedure fits easily into catheterization laboratory practice.
- The Galileo™ centering catheter is inflated with saline only.
- The centering catheter has a distal rapid exchange design. The guidewire should remain in place during the delivery of the radiation dose because it does not significantly affect the amount of radiation received by the target tissue.

Why I like the Galileo™ system

Beta-radiation
The use of ^{32}P, a beta-emitting isotope, minimizes exposure to the patient and to medical personnel. It allows for short dwell time and therefore minimal additional procedure time.

Centering
The centering catheter centers the source in the artery lumen even in curved segments (Figure 10.6). Centering of the radiation source is important, as it should allow the radiation dose to be delivered in a more uniform and controlled manner (Figure 10.7).

Perfusion
The helical design of the centering catheter is designed to allow for both distal and side branch perfusion during the delivery of the radiation dose (Figure 10.8). The perfusion capability may reduce the incidence of 'fractionation' or the delivery of the radiation dose in two distinct fractions, which in turn translates into a shorter procedure time.

Automatic, 'hands-off' delivery
Drawing from afterloader technology employed in radiation oncology, the Galileo™ source delivery unit automatically calculates the dwell time needed to deliver the correct radiation dose to the artery. Through the touch-screen display, the physician first advances an inactive 'dummy' or 'check' wire to ensure that the radiation path is clear, and then advances the active wire. The SDU automatically retracts the wire when the dose has been delivered, ensuring that the radiation source cannot be left in the artery for more than the prescribed time. Also, if the physician decides to retract the radiation source before the treatment is complete, the SDU will store the remaining treatment time so that the remaining dose can be automatically and precisely delivered.

Safety features
The Galileo™ system is designed with a number of safety features to reduce the possibility of any procedural safety problems. These include:

- An inactive 'dummy' wire to check the radiation path and to allow for delivery of the radiation dose to the correct location.
- An emergency stop button, an emergency back-up motor, and a manual retract mechanism.
- A force-sensing mechanism, which prevents the wire from being advanced with excessive force.

- A radioactive source that is sealed inside a wire and travels inside the sealed lumen of the centering catheter, providing a double radiation barrier.

Ease of operation

The Galileo™ system has been designed to fit with minimal impact into the practice of interventional cardiologists. The touch-screen display allows the entire procedure to be performed at the patient's bedside. The dosimetry is straightforward: the physician need only enter the reference lumen diameter and the SDU calculates the dwell time required to deliver the appropriate dose. The use of beta-radiation allows for a short procedure time and minimal exposure to catheterization laboratory personnel. The radiation source wire is exchanged through a safe, easy and fast procedure.

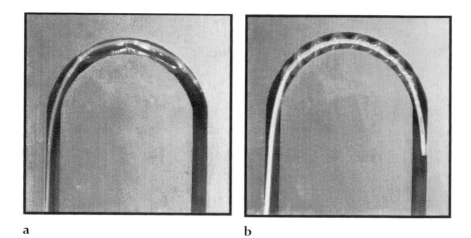

a   b

Figure 10.6 *Centering in a curved artery. (a) A simulated curve in the tube shows how a catheter without a centering mechanism lies eccentrically in the curved tube. (b) With the centering balloon inflated, the catheter is positioned in the center of the lumen of the curved tube. This centering mechanism assures a more uniform dose distribution to the target in the 'artery' wall.*

Synopsis of clinical trials

PREVENT

PREVENT (Proliferation REduction with Vascular ENergy Trial) was a feasibility trial designed to demonstrate the safety of the Guidant Galileo™

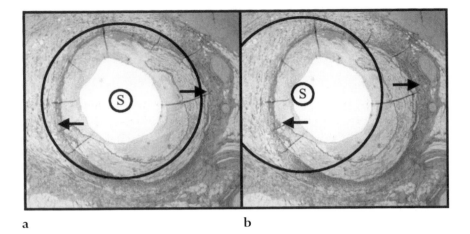

a   b

Figure 10.7 The importance of centering is illustrated in this figure. (a) The source
(S) is centered in a restenotic artery. The inner adventitia (arrows point to the EEL
indicating the border of media and adventitia) receives the prescribed dose of 20 Gy
indicated by the circle. (b) The source (S) is not centered, resulting in an excessively
high dose received by the adventitia on one side (left arrow) and an inadequately low
dose on the other side (right arrow).

intravascular radiotherapy system. Between November 1997 and May 1998, 72
patients were randomized to receive 0 (control), 16, 20 or 24 Gy to 1 mm
into the artery wall. Clinical sites included Baylor College of Medicine
(principal investigator (PI): A. Raizner), Stanford University (PI: S. Oesterle),
and Washington Heart Center (PI: R. Waksman). Of the 72 lesions treated, 47
(65%) were de novo and 25 (35%) were restenotic, including 21 (29%) in-
stent restenoses. PTCA alone was performed in 28 (39%) and a stent was
placed in 44 (61%). Follow-up angiography performed at 6 months revealed a
dramatic reduction of late loss index in the radiotherapy group compared with
control (5% versus 51%, $P = 0.0001$). Restenosis within the treated segment
of artery was 6% in the radiotherapy group compared with 33% in the
control group ($P = 0.015$), an 81% reduction. The primary clinical end-point
was major adverse cardiac events (MACE) defined as death, myocardial
infarction (MI) or TLR. MACE occurred in 16% of radiotherapy patients
compared with 24% of control patients. Radiation therapy was as effective in
patients treated with stents as it was in patients treated with balloon alone.
Additionally, no differences were observed among those who received 16, 20
or 24 Gy. Subgroup analysis of those treated for in-stent restenosis showed a
late loss index of only 9% and a TLR of 12% (which may be compared with a
historical control from the WRIST trial indicating a 65% late loss index and
64% TLR for in-stent restenosis patients).

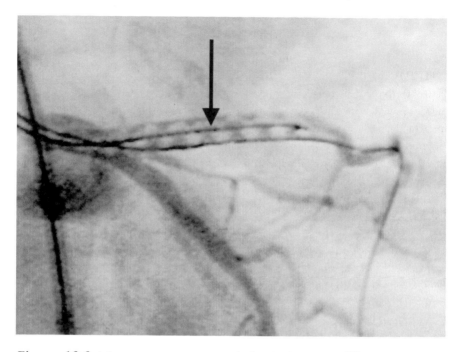

Figure 10.8 *A human coronary artery with the Guidant Galileo™ spiral balloon centering catheter positioned in the proximal left anterior descending. The criss-cross appearance indicates the pattern of flow through the spiral channels. There is excellent distal flow. Even though the proximal end of the balloon is in the left main, the spiral configuration allows for ample flow down the circumflex and a smaller branch of the left anterior descending. The arrow points to the inactive (dummy) source wire which is centered within the lumen.*

Thus, PREVENT was a positive trial demonstrating that intravascular radiotherapy with the Guidant Galileo™ system is safe as measured by MACE rates and the absence of untoward angiographic findings (e.g. aneurysms, non-healing dissections, etc). The method is feasible in arteries treated with either stents or PTCA alone, and in restenotic as well as de novo lesions. Further, radiation therapy was effective in significantly reducing restenosis within the radiation treatment zone, as measured by a low rate of restenosis and late lumen loss, in in-stent restenosis as well as in de novo lesions. The results of this pilot study support the need for larger randomized trials to substantiate the effectiveness of radiotherapy for reducing restenosis and clinical events.

PREVENT-CE
The PREVENT-CE trial is an ongoing parallel study to PREVENT being performed at five institutions worldwide. The trial design is identical to that

of PREVENT performed in the USA (see above). The anticipated total enrollment is 100 patients. The results of this study are expected in late 1999.

INHIBIT

INHIBIT (INtimal Hyperplasia Inhibition with Beta In-stent Trial) is a randomized, double-blind clinical trial using the Guidant Galileo™ intravascular radiotherapy system in the treatment of in-stent restenosis. Patients are randomized to receive 0 (control) or 20 Gy to 1 mm into the artery wall. The primary end-point of this trial is MACE (TLR, Q-wave MI or death) at 9 months. The first patient was enrolled in August 1998. This trial is expected to randomize 310 patients. The results of this trial are anticipated towards the end of 2000.

Several additional trials are planned to investigate the safety and efficacy of the Galileo™ system and a number of other clinical indications, including small vessel disease and saphenous vein grafts.

11. Boston Scientific/SCIMED Intravascular Radiation System

*Cardiology Center and *Division of Radiation Oncology, University Hospital, Geneva, Switzerland*

Vitali E Verin and Youri G Popowski*

Definition	The Boston Scientific/SCIMED intravascular radiation system comprises: • ^{90}Y pure beta-emitting linear source • introducer catheter allowing intra-arterial centering of the source • automated afterloader.

History	• **December 1992** Verin and Popowski propose to Schneider (Europe) AG the concept of intra-arterial beta-irradiation • **1993** Schneider develops the first centering catheter for beta-irradiation • **June 1994** Experiment with hypercholesterolemic rabbits (Geneva) • **June–November 1995** Clinical pilot study (Geneva) • September 1996 6 months' toxicity study in rabbits (Lyon) • **1996** Sauerwein develops the first automatic afterloader for beta-brachytherapy • **January 1997** Long-term efficacy and safety study in a pig model (Groton) • **July 1997** Efficacy study in an overstretch and stent injury model in a pig (R Waksman, Washington) • **September 1997** Start of the European Multicenter Clinical Dose-Finding Study • **1998** Schneider is acquired by Boston Scientific Corporation • **August 1999** Successful results of the European Multi-center Clinical Dose-Finding Study reported at CESF (Barcelona, Spain)

Technical specifications (Figure 11.1)

Source	
Design	Flexible coil affixed at the end of a thrust wire between proximal and distal tungsten markers
Diameter	0.34 mm (0.014 inch)
Length	29 mm
Material	Titanium-coated pure yttrium
Y–Ti wire diameter	0.1 mm (0.004 inch)
Isotope:	^{90}Y
Mode of decay	beta
Decay energy	2.284 MeV
Half-life	64.1 hours
Max activity	150 mCi
Centering catheter	
Design	Segmented balloon consisting of four interconnected compartments
Available diameters	2.5, 3.0, 3.5, 4.0 mm
Balloon length	25 mm
Minimal guiding catheter lumen	0.064 inch (compatible with 6 Fr guidings)
Inflation media	Contrast, CO_2
Afterloading machine comprises	
Supporting system:	
serving and controlling computer	
software allowing dummy and source motion control	
protocol printer	
power supply unit	
Afterloader:	
source container	
dummy container	
radiation shield	
dummy/source drive system	

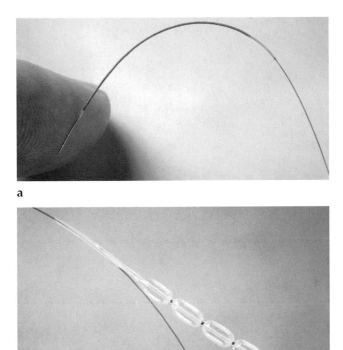

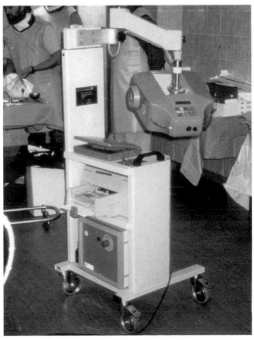

Figure 11.1 (a) Yttrium coil fixed on the distal end of a thrust wire. The coil is made of titanium-coated pure yttrium wire. (b) Centering catheter. The four interconnecting chambers allow centering of the source lumen relative to the arterial lumen. Note the 20-mm long distal tip of this device ensuring its 'monorail' introduction and the three radiopaque platinum markers situated at sites of balloon waists. (c) Afterloader with its support.

a

b

c

97

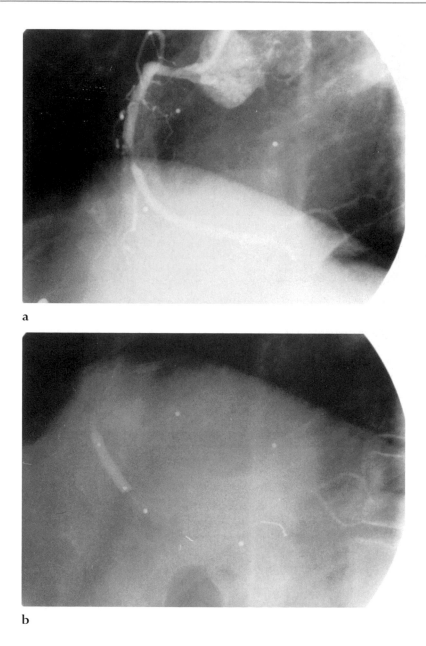

a

b

Figure 11.2 Endoluminal beta-irradiation of right coronary artery. Left anterior oblique view. (a) Tight RCA stenosis. (b) PTCA with 3.5-mm balloon. (c) Intracoronary irradiation procedure. The four compartments of the centering catheter are inflated with contrast medium. The beta-emitting ^{90}Y source is situated inside the centering catheter. Note that the length of the radioactive segment is delimited by two radiopaque tungsten markers. The centering balloon radiopaque waists confirm the correct centering of the ^{90}Y source inside the artery. (d) Good immediate angiographic result of PTCA-irradiation procedure.

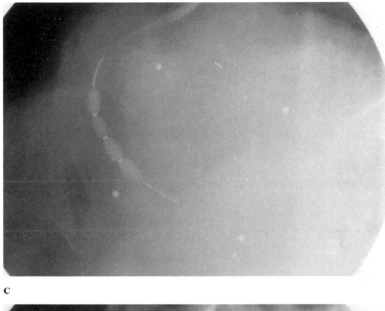

c

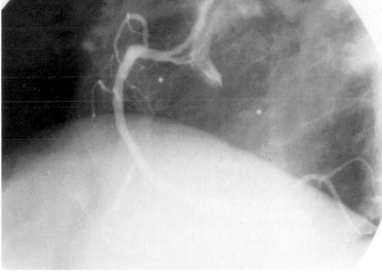

d

Tips and tricks

During the animal experiments and the clinical studies the centering catheter and radiation source showed excellent mechanical properties (pushability, trackability) and ease of handling. Computerized afterloader was extremely reliable and user-friendly. We feel that almost all lesions accessible for conventional percutaneous transluminal coronary angioplasty (PTCA) could be accessed and irradiated with this system.

Indications for use

- Any de novo lesion undergoing PTCA with or without stenting
- Restenotic lesions after PTCA with or without stent

Why I like the Boston Scientific/SCIMED system

1. It provides all advantages related to use of the beta source in comparison with conventional gamma:
   - markedly steeper dose decline in tissue, hence significantly lower undue irradiation of surrounding periarterial structures
   - much lower radioprotection problems making the system use compatible with standard catheterization laboratory conditions; no additional protection is required
   - possibility of a high focal dose delivery in a relatively short time interval.
2. Good trackability of the centering device and high flexibility of the ^{90}Y coiled source allows the system to be used even in a very tortuous coronary anatomy.
3. Centering of the radioactive source relative to the arterial lumen allows uniform intramural dose distribution. Expected effect: homogeneous inhibition of neointimal hyperplasia.
4. Sealed source lumen of the centering device prevents contact of the source with body fluids.
5. Radiopaque markers make positioning of the centering device and delivery of the radioactive source very easy.
6. The automated afterloader makes dose delivery user-friendly and provides for an important degree of safety and security for radiation protection.

Distinguishing features of the afterloader

- Fully automated irradiation protocol
- Automated advancement and positioning of the source
- Dedicated dummy source to check friction and to determine exact position
- Easy, quick and safe exchange of the source
- Automatic compensation for source decay

Synopsis of clinical trials

1. June 1995 – May 1996: Clinical pilot study (Figure 11.2)
   - Purpose: to study feasibility and safety of intracoronary irradiation
   - Number of patients: 15
   - Non-randomized, non-comparative
   - Single-center (University Hospital of Geneva)
2. September 1997 – August 1999: Dose-finding clinical study
   - Purpose: to determine the effect of various doses of beta-radiation on post-PTCA restenosis
   - Number of patients: 160
   - Randomized
   - Prospective
   - Multi-center (five European centers)

NB! This system is in a development phase and not yet commercially available.

12. THE RE-RADCATH™ SYSTEM

CVRT Ltd/Soreq, Yavne, Israel

Efi Lavie, Danny Kijel, Eli Sayag, Rosanna Chan and Ron
Waksman

Definition	The Re-RadCath™ is a radioactive catheter for the treatment of restenosis. The source is a 186/188 rhenium solid coil. It is mainly a beta source. The system has four components: a radioactive catheter containing a flexible coil, a test ('dummy') catheter, a shielded containment device, and a closed-end lumen delivery catheter (Figures 12.1 and 12.2).

History	• **1997**	The concept of Re irradiation and assembly was developed at Soreq nuclear research center
	• **1997–98**	First animal trials at the Washington Hospital Center (Figure 12.3). The model was an overstretched balloon injury in pigs
	• **1999**	IDE application

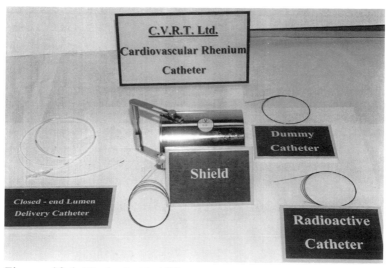

Figure 12.1 *The Re-RadCath™ system.*

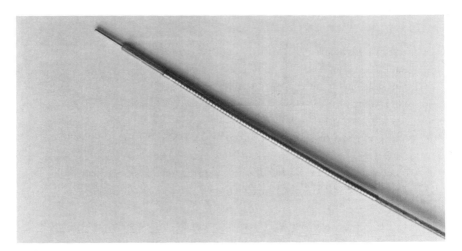

Figure 12.2 *Close-up microscope picture of the Re coil. Note that the ribbon pitches are adjacent to one another.*

Technical specifications (Figures 12.4 and 12.5)	
Physical design	32-mm long flexible coil made of natural rhenium metal
Source diameter	0.85 mm (0.033 inch)
Encapsulation	The source is sealed in a polymer capsule
Catheter	Polyimide
Isotope	Re-186 and Re-188
Half-life	90 hours and 17 hours respectively
Radiation	Mainly beta, maximal energy 1.07 MeV for Re-186 and 2.1 MeV for Re-188
Shield	Lucite and lead; shield weight ~ 14 kg
Source fluoroscopic visibility	Excellent
Activity	Post-production: ~ 3 Ci for Re-188 and 700 mCi for Re-186
Prescription dose	15 Gy at 2 mm from the source center
Treatment time	3–6 min

Tips and tricks

- The non-radioactive test wire is inserted into the sterile delivery catheter.
- The delivery catheter is positioned over a flexible 0.014-inch wire at the lesion.
- The non-radioactive wire is withdrawn.
- The radioactive Re source is manually pushed into the delivery catheter.
- Fluoroscopic visualization verifies the position of the source.
- The source is left for a time period sufficient to deliver the assigned dose (3–6 min).
- The treatment can be stopped at any time.
- The source is non-centered; however, the delivery catheter acts as a spacer.
- The Re source is retracted manually back to the shielded containment device.

Indications for clinical use

- Recurrent restenosis
- In-stent restenosis

Why I like the Re-RadCath™ system

- Use of beta source—less hazardous to patient and medical staff
- Capability to treat several patients
- Short treatment time (< 10 min)
- Short half-life—easy waste management
- Manual, precise and convenient delivery catheter
- Compact and low weight shielded containment device
- Radiopaque source enables accurate guiding and positioning of the source

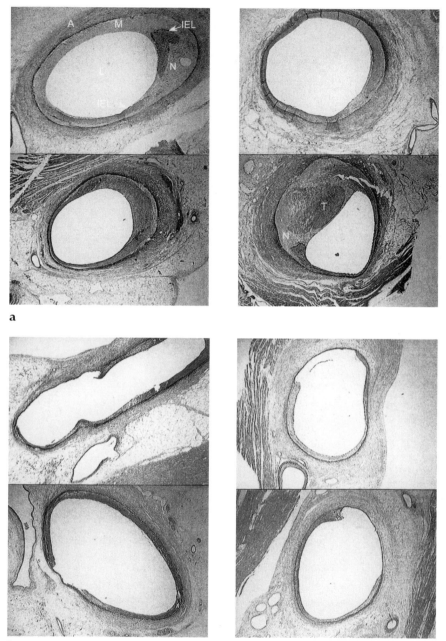

Figure 12.3 *Histology results from an animal study.*
(a) Control non-irradiated artery (A: adventitia; IEL: internal elastic lamina; L: lumen; M: media; N: neointima; T: thrombus);
(b) The radiation effect of a 15-Gy dose on neointima formation.

106

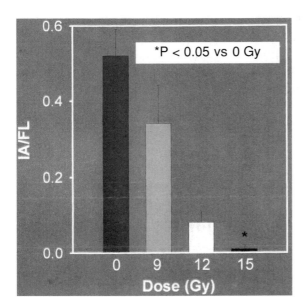

Figure 12.4 The
dose–response effect.
Increasing the dose
induced a decrease of the
IA/FL ratio. IA: intimal
area (mm^2); FL: medial
fracture length (mm).

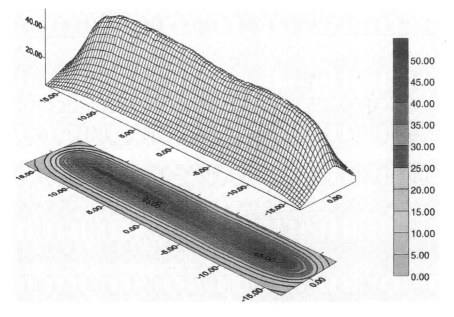

Figure 12.5 Film dosimetry study. Re-188/186 wire dose distribution curve 68 h
after production (depth = 2.4 mm). The longitudinal source uniformity is shown and
the lateral variation of the dose vs distance from the source is demonstrated.

107

On-going and planned clinical trials

- Clinical trials are planned to start before the end of 1999 in several centers in Israel
- IDE applied for a clinical trial in the WA Hospital Center in 1999
- Multicenter trials are planned in Europe during the year 2000

Results from the animal studies

Using the porcine coronary model, eight pigs underwent balloon overstretch (BI) injury to 16 coronary arteries. Following the BI, a 30-mm in length radioactive Re-188/186 coiled-wire (1-mm in diameter) was introduced to cover the angioplasty site in eight of the injuried arteries. The prescribed dose was 15 Gy delivered to a distance of 2 into the artery wall, and the dose rate varied from 9–2 Gy/min. Two weeks after the procedure the animals were killed, the arteries were perfusion fixed, stained, and examained by histological and morphometric techniques. Results showed complete inhibition of neointima formation in the irradiated arteries, regardless to the difference in the dose rate. There was no excess of thrombus, fibrin, or fibrosis in the irradiated arteries compared to control. Intracoronary delivery of the radioactive coiled Re-188/186 is feasible, safe, and results with consistent homogenous inhibition of neointima formation in the porcine model.

13. THE RADIOACTIVE STENT

Isostent, Inc., Belmont, CA, USA

Tim A Fischell, David R Fischell, Christoph Hehrlein and Robert E Fischell

Definition/ Description	A balloon-expandable or self-expanding stent rendered radioactive by activation in a cyclotron or by ion implantation with beta-particle emitting and/or gamma-emitting radioisotope, for the purpose of inhibiting neointimal hyperplasia and restenosis after stenting of arterial, venous or other tubular structures (Figure 13.1).

History		
	• **December 1989**	Concept of a radioactive stent for the prevention of restenosis proposed by Fischell et al
	• **1993–97**	Experimental studies from Europe and the USA provided proof of principle with selected activities of ^{32}P
	• **7 October, 1996**	First radioisotope stent implanted in coronary circulation at Borgess Medical Center, Kalamazoo, MI, USA
	• **1996–1998**	Clinical evaluation of this device in the coronary circulation at very low stent activities (0.5–1.5 μCi) with Palmaz–Schatz™ stent design
	• **1998–present**	Clinical evaluation of this device at higher stent activities (1.5–20.0 μCi) with Palmaz–Schatz™ and newer BX stent™ design
	• **1999–present**	Testing of cold- and hot-end stents to resolve issues of 'edge restenosis'

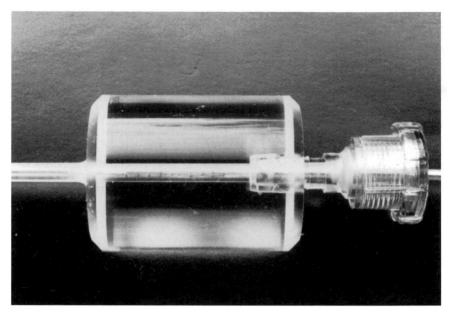

a

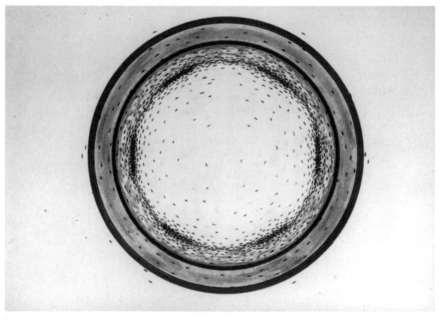

b

Figure 13.1 (a) ^{32}P radioactive stent mounted on the stent delivery system and covered with a protective lucite plastic shield to prevent radiation exposure to the operator. (b) Schematic illustrates the localized emission of beta particles (electrons) from the stent struts.

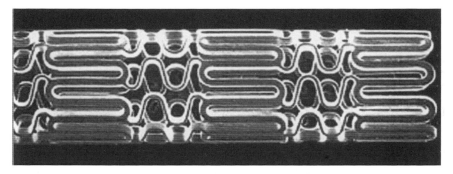

Figure 13.2 Newer generation BX stent™ for possible future radioisotope applications.

Technical specifications

- Radioisotope used: ^{32}P at present. Other isotopes under development, including gamma emitter palladium-103
- Current method for making stent radioactive: ion implantation
- Range of activities tested in clinical setting: 0.5–20.0 μCi of ^{32}P (on 15 mm stent), 25 mm stent with 6–20 μCi ^{32}P
- Conformity with existing stent manufacturing guidelines
- Uniform distribution of the radioisotope (< 5% deviation)
- Leeching of the radioisotope should be negligible (< 1% for the life of the stent)
- Stent delivered with lucite shield to protect operator from beta particle irradiation during stent implantation

Tips and tricks

The techniques used for implantation of a radioactive stent are nearly identical to those required for optimal placement of a non-radioactive balloon-expandable stent. Lucite shield (over stent) is inserted into standard Tuohy–Borst connector at the proximal end of the guiding catheter and will protect the operator from radiation exposure during stent implantation. The radioactive stent should be implanted to cover the entire length of the lesion. Recent data from the Milan experience with Dr A Colombo suggest that care needs to be taken to minimize barotrauma beyond the stent edges during stent implantation. This may be more feasible by implanting the BX stent™ using a direct stenting technique with a balloon to artery ratio of ≤ 1.1.

Indications for clinical use

- De novo native coronary lesions
- Restenosis lesions
- Saphenous vein graft lesions
- Future uses may include peripheral artery stenting, biliary stenting, prostate stenting, bronchial and esophageal stenting

Why I like the radioactive stent

The technique of implanting a ^{32}P radioactive stent is essentially identical to that of a non-radioactive stent. A radioactive stent delivers endovascular radiation locally to the target lesion without significant additional radiation exposure to the operator or catheterization laboratory personnel. It allows the use of very low activity devices compared with catheter-based brachytherapy systems (e.g. 3.0–20.0 μCi for ^{32}P radioactive stent versus 30 000–500 000 μCi for brachytherapy catheters). Once safety and efficacy can be established, the beta-particle emitting radioactive stents should be the safest and most efficient method for prescribing endovascular irradiation.

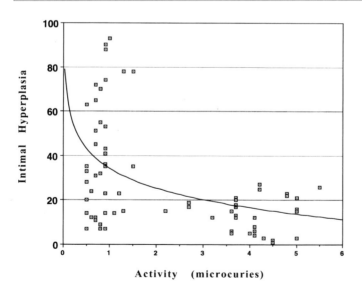

Figure 13.3 Scattergram showing the in-stent neointimal volume, as measured by IVUS, at 6 months. These data compare the original low activity (0.5–1.5 μCi) cohort and the 3–6 μCi cohort from the Milan experience (data kindly provided by Dr N Weissman, Georgetown University, IVUS core laboratory). Data show a dose-dependent decrease in within-stent neointima with a ^{32}P radioisotope stent (P < 0.001).

112

Current and planned clinical trials

- Clinical and angiographic follow-up of 28 patients (Milan) with higher activity BX stents, implanted using 'gentle technique' with balloon to artery ratio ~1.1:1. Six-month follow-ups to be complete by October 1999.
- European trial of cold-end stents using 25-mm length with only central 15 mm containing radioisotope. Trial started June 1999.
- Pilot trial of hot-end stents on new balloon delivery system to minimize edge trauma. Trial scheduled to start by late 1999.

Review of current literature

Despite improvements in long-term outcomes following intracoronary stent placement, restenosis remains a significant problem, particularly in long lesions and vessels with smaller diameters.[1,2] Experimental and clinical data have demonstrated that in-stent restenosis is principally caused by neointimal formation.[3-6] Endovascular radiation has been proposed as a method to reduce neointimal formation and thus prevent in-stent restenosis.[7-15]

Catheter-based intravascular brachytherapy with the gamma-emitting radioisotope Ir-192 has been shown to be effective in the reduction of neointimal hyperplasia in the treatment of restenosis in three placebo-controlled clinical trials.[12,15] While these studies established the clinical efficacy of endovascular irradiation to prevent restenosis, the impracticalities and safety issues related to the use of a gamma source may limit the acceptance of this therapy. Alternatively, we have proposed the use of a stent as the platform for local radiation delivery as a means to prevent restenosis.

Low-dose beta-particle irradiation inhibits smooth muscle proliferation and migration in vitro.[13] Experimental studies have demonstrated that stents ion implanted with ^{32}P reduce neointimal formation at activities as low as 0.14 μCi.[7,8,10,14] The purpose of this summary is to review the current status of radioactive stents for the prevention of in-stent restenosis.

Stent dosimetry

The dosimetry of a ^{32}P stent has previously been described in detail. Janicki et al characterized the near field dose of a 1.0-μCi 15-mm length Palmaz–Schatz

(Cordis, Johnson and Johnson Co., Warren, NJ, USA) using a modification of the dose-point-kernel method.[16] Modification of the dose distribution around a uniform cylinder of ^{32}P to account for the geometry of a tubular slotted Palmaz–Schatz stent with mathematical modeling, allowed construction of three-dimensional dose maps. For a 1.0-μCi 15-mm length ^{32}P stent, at a distance of 0.1 mm, dose values of $\approx$2500 cGy are delivered at the strut wires (peaks) and $\approx$800 cGy between the wires (valleys) over one half-life (14.3 days) (Figure 13.2). The non-uniformity of dosing reflective of the stent geometry decreases at distances of 1–2 mm from the surface. The dosimetry predicted by the dose calculations correlated well with the measured dose using radiochromic film. While these data provide an in vitro analysis of dosing from a radioactive stent, the actual dose distribution will be affected by variations in atherosclerotic plaque morphology and the symmetry of stent expansion.

Safety issues

The use of beta-particle-emitting radioisotope stents should be one of the safest and the simplest means of administering intravascular brachytherapy. With ^{32}P, it is expected that the stent activities required to achieve therapeutic effects in human atherosclerotic vessels will be in the 3.0–25 μCi range. As such, this radioactivity is approximately 10 000–30 000 times lower than the radioactivity of beta-catheter systems and a 20 000–170 000 times lower activity than currently used gamma-emitting catheter sources. The use of such a low activity beta source ensures that there is significantly less risk of mishandling, loss or embolization. Using beta-irradiation only, the source is easily shielded (see Figure 13.1) and provides minimal risks for catherization laboratory personnel handling the device. The estimated maximal dose to critical organs for a patient receiving a 25-μCi ^{32}P stent would be < 2.5 mRem, which is approximately 1/500th of the dose to critical organs from an average x-ray dose using fluoroscopy during coronary angioplasty. The relatively short half-life of ^{32}P ensures that the radioactivity of the stent will be reduced to background levels within 4–5 months after implantation.

Early clinical experience with radioisotope stents

The initial clinical experience with beta-particle-emitting stents began in October 1996. The Phase I Isostent for Restenosis Intervention Study (IRIS) was a non-randomized trial designed to evaluate the safety of implanting very low activity (0.5–1.0 μCi) ^{32}P 15-mm length Palmaz–Schatz coronary stents in patients with symptomatic de novo or restenosis native coronary lesions. The enrollment for this trial was completed on January 14, 1997 with 32 patients receiving a beta-particle-emitting stent.

In this feasibility trial, stent placement was successful in all patients. The mean stent activity at the time of implant in the IRIS trial was 0.7 μCi. There were no cases of subacute stent thrombosis, target lesion revascularization, death or other major cardiac events within the first 30 days (primary safety end-point), thus, demonstrating acceptable early event-free survival. At the 6-month follow-up there was a binary restenosis rate of 31% (10/32) and a clinically driven target vessel revascularization (TVR) rate of 21%. Interestingly, there was only one restenosis (proximal to stent) out of the 10 patients treated for restenosis lesions (10%) and only 18% for patients receiving stents > 0.75 μCi. There were no further TVR events between 6 months and 24 months. Of note, in the de novo subgroup, the mean reference vessel diameter was 2.85 mm, and 7/22 reference vessels in this subgroup were < 2.50 mm. One stent was implanted in a vessel with a reference vessel size of 1.95 mm.

Quantitative angiographic follow up at 6 months demonstrated a lesional late loss of 0.94 mm for the group as a whole, and 0.70 mm for the restenosis subgroup. These data are similar to late loss data from contemporary stent trials with non-radioactive stents. The Phase I IRIS trial (1B) was a second low-dose extension of the trial to test the safety of higher activity (0.75–1.5 mCi) stents at five additional medical centers in the USA. Twenty-five patients were enrolled in this extension of the Phase I trial. The mean stent activity was 1.14 μCi at the time of implantation. All 25 cases were implanted successfully, without reported serious adverse events at 1-month safety follow-up. The restenosis rate (32%) and late loss data were similar to the 1A results. A small safety trial with 1.5–3.0 μCi 15-mm length ^{32}P stents was also performed in Heidelberg, Germany and Rotterdam in The Netherlands. To date, approximately 30 of these stents have been implanted successfully. There were no adverse events noted in this group at the 30-day safety end-point. Restenosis data at these lower activities also did not suggest a significant beneficial effect.

Based upon human smooth muscle cell experiments looking at the effects of continuous low dose-rate beta-irradiation, it was determined that the likely effective stent activity for de novo coronary lesions should be in the 3.0–25.0 μCi range (IRIS 1A mean activity was 0.7 μCi). It should be noted that in some animal models the effective activity was as high as 26 μCi for a 15-mm long, 3.0-mm diameter ^{32}P stent.[10] It is possible that a lower stent activity could be effective in restenosis lesions if the proliferating target tissue derives from the recently formed neointima rather than the adventitia, as is likely for de novo lesions.

Milan studies

Approximately 200 ^{32}P stents with activities ranging between 1.5 and 20.0 μCi
have been implanted in Milan by Dr Antonio Colombo and his colleagues.
There were no major adverse cardiac events (MACE; death, MI,
revascularization) events reported at 30 days in this higher activity cohort.
There has been one reported late subacute thrombosis (i.e. ≤0.5% overall
SAT rate). This one SAT occurred in a patient who had received three stents
and was medically non-compliant with antiplatelet medications. Thus the early
safety of these implants appears to be quite good, particularly when compared
with recent reports of relatively high SAT rates in catheter-based radiation
treatment patients who received a non-radioactive stent. Late follow-up data
from these higher activity cohorts has demonstrated a dose-dependent
reduction of neointimal hyperplasia within the stent. If lesion restenosis rates
were reported for within the stent only, as has been used in trials such as the
BERT feasibility trial, the restenosis rate in the patients with stent activities
≥ 3.0 mCi was ≤ 10%. However, in these higher activity stents there appears
to be some increased restenosis at or beyond the stent edges. This has been
referred to as the 'candy wrapper', characterized as a widely patent middle
zone, but with narrowing at one or both edges. The overall incidence of the
edge effect restenosis varied in the Milan cohort from ∼ 35% to as high as
55%. In this series, edge barotrauma as predicted by a high balloon to artery
ratio (B/A ratio) at the time of implant appeared to be a significant predictor
of this edge restenosis. The B/A ratio in the cohort without edge narrowing
was 1.09, versus 1.22 in the group with edge restenosis ($P < 0.05$).

Future directions

Stent restenosis often occurs in the mid-stent at the site of the central
articulation of the 15-mm length Palmaz–Schatz (P–S) stent.[3] To eliminate
problems of dose fall off in the central articulation zone of the P–S stent, all
recent and future radioisotope stent implants are now performed with the
BX™ stent platform. The first generation BX™ (Isostent Inc., San Carlos,
CA, USA) is a novel stainless steel balloon-expandable stent designed without
a central articulation. The BX™ has honeycomb-shaped cells linked by
alternating articulation geometry that provides longitudinal flexibility while
maintaining the radial strength of the stent. The uniform geometry of the
BX™ appears to have a favorable effect on the dose distribution for a ^{32}P
stent. The difference between maximal and minimal near field tissue dose of
irradiation is less for the BX™ than the Palmaz–Schatz design.

116

Future clinical trials are now focusing upon the issue of edge restenosis. In Milan 28 patients had intermediate activity ^{32}P stents implanted using the original SDS balloon, but a more gentle implantation technique. The focus of this series was to implant the stents with a low B/A ratio and try to avoid barotrauma outside the stent margins. Since at least part of the edge restenosis appears to be related to negative late remodeling, a small clinical trial has been initiated using 25-mm stents with cold ends (no ^{32}P on the proximal and distal 5 mm of the stent). It is hoped that this may yield a similar reduction of neointimal hyperplasia within the stent body while eliminating any potential stimulatory effects outside the stent margins. To date $\sim$ 20 implants have been performed, and early and late results are pending. Another, more promising, approach involves the use of a new high-pressure stent delivery balloon with ≤ 1.5 mm of balloon overhang past the stent edges, combined with stents that have more ^{32}P on the distal and proximal stent edges. It is hoped that this approach (hot ends with minimal overhang) may yield better dosing and less trauma in the critical 1–2 mm at the proximal and distal stent margins. This pilot trial should start by the end of 1999.

Other dosing strategies are also possible with alternative radioisotopes, including gamma emitters, and/or longer acting beta emitters, or even a combination of radioisotopes on the same stent. A self-expanding stent platform may be used in conjunction with radioisotope for peripheral applications and as a means to minimize or even eliminate barotrauma at the stent edges at the time of stent implantation.

Conclusions

Recent clinical studies suggest that catheter-based intravascular radiation therapy may be effective in the prevention of restenosis. The early clinical results with more than 250 clinical implants of low activity ^{32}P Palmaz–Schatz and BX^{TM} radioactive stents have demonstrated excellent procedural and 30-day event-free survival. Encouraging data have also been collected demonstrating a potent dose-dependent reduction of neointimal hyperplasia within the stent, using 15-mm length stents containing 3–20 μCi of ^{32}P. Further safety and efficacy pilot trials are ongoing in 1999 to try to eliminate the edge restenosis problem observed in the early series of patients using higher activity stents. Implementation of a large-scale randomized clinical trial will commence if and when these trials suggest a beneficial therapeutic effect from this technology. Thus, future studies will continue to focus upon optimal stent design, low barotrauma implants and alternative dosing strategies.

Acknowledgments

We gratefully acknowledge the contributions to this work by Dr Antonio Colombo, Dr Patrick Serruys, C. Janicki, the IRIS investigators, the angiographic and IVUS core labs and Isostent, Inc.

References

1. Serruys PW, De Jaegere P, Kiemeneij F et al. for the Benestent Study Group. A comparison of balloon-expandable-stent implantation with balloon angioplasty in patients with coronary artery disease. *N Engl J Med* 1994; **331**:489–495.

2. Fischman DL, Leon MB, Baim DS et al. for the Stent Restenosis Study Investigators. A randomized comparison of coronary-stent placement and balloon angioplasty in the treatment of coronary artery disease. *N Engl J Med* 1994; **331**:496–501.

3. Painter JA, Mintz GS, Wong SC et al. Serial intravascular ultrasound studies fail to show evidence of chronic Palmaz–Schatz stent recoil. *Am J Cardiol* 1995; **75**:398–400.

4. Hoffmann R, Mintz G, Dussaillant G et al. Patterns and mechanisms of in-stent restenosis: a serial intravascular ultrasound study. *Circulation* 1996; **94**:1247–1254.

5. Edelman ER, Rogers C. Hoop dreams: stents without restenosis. *Circulation* 1996; **94**:1199–1202.

6. Serruys PW, Kutryk JB. The state of the stent: current practices, controversies, and future trends. *Am J Cardiol* 1996; **78(suppl 3A)**: 4–7.

7. Laird JR, Carter AJ, Kufs W et al. Inhibition of neointimal proliferation with a Beta particle emitting stent. *Circulation* 1996; **93**:529–536.

8. Carter AJ, Laird JR, Bailey LR et al. The effects of endovascular radiation from a β-particle emitting stent in a porcine restenosis model: a dose response study. *Circulation* 1996; **94**:2364–2368.

9. Hehrlein, C, Gollan C, Dönges K et al. Low-dose radioactive endovascular stents prevent smooth muscle cell proliferation and neointimal hyperplasia in rabbits. *Circulation* 1995; **92**:1570–1575.

10. Hehrlein, C, Stintz M, Kinscherf R et al. Pure β-particle emitting stents inhibit neointima formation in rabbits. *Circulation* 1996; **93**:641–645.

11. Waksman R, Robinson KA, Crocker IR et al. Intracoronary radiation before stent implantation inhibits neointima formation in stented canine coronary arteries. *Circulation* 1995; **92**:1383–1386.

12. Tierstein PS, Massullo V, Jani S et al. Catheter-based radiotherapy to inhibit restenosis after coronary stenting. *N Engl J Med* 1997; **96**:727–732.

13. Fischell TA, Kharma BK, Fischell DR et al. Low-dose, β-particle emission from stent wire results in complete, localized inhibition of smooth muscle cell proliferation. *Circulation* 1994; **90**:2956–2963.

14. Rivard A, Leclerc G, Bouchard M et al. Low-dose β-emitting radioactive stents inhibit neointimal hyperplasia in porcine coronary arteries; an histological assessment. *J Am Coll Cardiol* 1997; **29**:238A.

15. Waksman R, Laird JR, Benenati J et al. Intravascular radiation therapy for patients with in-stent restenosis: 6-month follow-up of a randomized clinical study (abstract). *Circulation* 1998; **98**:I-651:3721

16. Janicki C, Duggan DM Coffey CW, Fischell DR, Fischell TA. Radiation dose from a phosphorous-32 impregnated wire mesh vascular stent. *Med Phys* 1997; **24**:437–445.

14. SOLUTION-APPLIED BETA-EMITTING RADIOISOTOPE (CURE) SYSTEM

Columbia University, New York, NY, USA

Judah Weinberger

Definition	Intravascular radiation delivery system consisting of a beta-emitting radiopharmaceutical, in solution, as a vehicle to inflate a balloon catheter at a vascular target site.

Brief history of the device

Various approaches to delivery of intravascular radiation have been proposed based on removable sources, and modeled on radiation delivery systems from brachytherapy for malignant processes. These have, generally, involved the use of high-activity gamma emitters. Because beta emitters deposit a large fraction of their energy locally, these isotopes have substantial safety advantages for both the operator and the patient over the gamma emitters. Efforts to make use of beta radioisotopes in solution awaited the development of an appropriate compound with an adequate biodistribution profile to deal safely with the rare intravascular release of the radioisotope-containing liquid. Building upon studies of the biodistribution of certain chelates of the rare earth rhenium, it has been possible to develop the current device for vascular radiation delivery. (See Figures 14.1–14.3.) Recent investigators have suggested that potassium perchlorate could be used to block thyroid uptake of non-chelated ^{188}Re as an alternative to other chelation approaches.

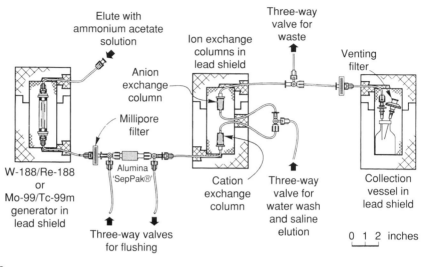

a

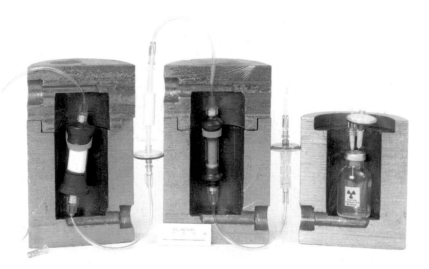

b

Figure 14.1 *Radiopharmaceutical preparation apparatus. (a) Schematic diagram of the set-up of the alumina-based tungsten-188/rhenium-188 generator system housed in a 2.5-cm thick lead shield attached to cartridge concentration system for concentration of the generator eluant. (b) Cut-away view of actual set-up.*

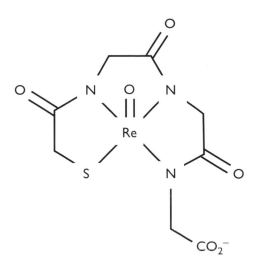

Figure 14.2 *Structure of* $^{188}Re\text{-}MAG_3$.

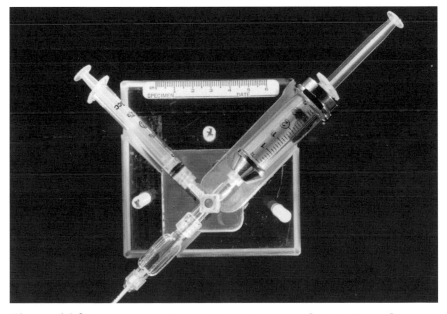

Figure 14.3 *Intracoronary radiation delivery device: a perfusion balloon inflation hub attached to a Lucite-shielded syringe containing* $^{188}Re\text{-}MAG_3$. *The additional syringe delivers contrast for mixing. The entire proximal balloon inflation structure is embedded in a Lucite–lead shield (shown here in cut-away view).*

Tips and tricks

- Co-ordinate your treatment with the radiation physicist, radiopharmacist, radiation oncologist, and radiation safety officer.
- Use plastic-backed absorbent towels covering a dedicated work area in the catheterization laboratory.
- For treatment in conjunction with balloon angioplasty, obtain a final angiographic result of less than 30% residual stenosis. If stent placement is contemplated, radiation treatment should be carried out after predilatation, but before stent deployment.
- Exchange for a *new* perfusion balloon (the treatment balloon) that has not undergone a negative prep. The balloon portion of the prep is done with the balloon positioned in the target coronary segment.
- Verify (preferably with the manufacturer) that the three-way stopcock will not leak when pressurized with the radioactive fluid.
- The length of the treatment balloon should be at least 4 mm longer than the dilating balloon or stent on each end. Inflate the balloon with ^{188}Re solution diluted with contrast (we use 50% Hypaque final).
- Remove the balloon, with the inflation device still attached, directly from the catheterization table into the radioactive waste bin.
- For a given dose of radiation, the time of irradiation is related to the activity of the ^{188}Re in the balloon. In a large artery, with no significant side branches in the treatment segment, perfusion balloon inflations of 5–10 min are usually well tolerated. If a major side branch originates from an arterial segment in the treatment volume, inflation times of 1–3 min are usually tolerated.

Proposed indications for use

This device will be studied for efficacy in preventing restenosis after de novo balloon angioplasty or together with stent implantation in native coronary and bypass lesions, as well as restenotic lesions after these procedures. Patients in whom an adequate angiographic result after intervention cannot be obtained should not be treated. Based upon efficacy information to be derived from multi-center trials, specific recommendations will be made.

Why I like the beta-emitting radioisotope system

Catheter-based radiotherapy with a beta-emitting radioisotope-filled balloon provides a technically simple, safe, and inexpensive means to deliver a radiation field that conforms to the vessel geometry in an optimal fashion. Centering of the balloon within the available lumens occurs during balloon inflation. Even when the vessel makes an angle, the balloon, and thus the source, conforms to the turn. These two features ensure the optimal field distribution obtainable from an intraluminal device. Finally, radiation disposal involves a simple quarantine of the radioactive device for 10 days, until the isotope has decayed, followed by standard 'red-bag' disposal.

Synopsis of ongoing and planned clinical trials

A single-center safety trial is currently under way at Columbia Presbyterian Medical Center using a ^{188}Re-MAG$_3$ solution to treat patients with clinically significant lesions of the native coronary system that are less than 30 mm long. Either de novo or restenotic lesions are eligible. A total of 40 patients are to be enrolled in this study, whose primary end-point is 30-day major cardiac events (death, target lesion revascularization, or myocardial infarction). Double-blind trials of this technique for delivery of brachytherapy are currently underway in Australia and in Korea.

Review of currently published literature

A large body of animal investigation and a more limited number of clinical studies have established the ability of ionizing radiation to inhibit vascular smooth muscle cell proliferation associated with restenosis. Human studies have reported that intravascular gamma-radiation inhibits a second restenosis event, after a first recurrence.[1] Studies using an encapsulated beta-emitting source, ^{90}Sr/^{90}Y, have suggested that this modality of radiation delivery may also be efficacious in humans (BERT trial). Thus the focus of developments in this area has been both the establishment of efficacy in larger groups, as well as optimization of a radiation delivery system.

Two of the most controversial issues surrounding intravascular radiation delivery involve the preference of beta- or gamma-emitting radioisotope sources, and the importance and value of source-centering in the artery. The relative importance of centering of intravascular radiation sources has been pointed out by our group.[2] Malcentering of a catheter-based solid source by as little as 0.5 mm could lead to errors in dosing of as much as fivefold. These errors are considerably worse for beta emitters than for gamma emitters. Such errors could lead to significant under- and overdosing with varying fractions of the vessel circumference. The clinical importance of this effect is not known.

Among the possible methods of delivering endovascular radiation, catheter-based encapsulated solid-source technologies will require a dedicated radiation delivery device. In an effort to obviate the necessity for additional hardware, and simultaneously take advantage of the considerable skills already present in the armamentarium of invasive cardiologists, use of a conventional balloon catheter to deliver a liquid isotope was an appealing possibility. The hurdles to be overcome in this approach are the minimization of the likelihood of contamination of patients and the catheterization laboratory, the safe handling of liquid radioisotopes, and a safe radiopharmaceutical to deal with inevitable balloon leakage or rupture, allowing systemic release of the radioisotope.

The effects of released radioisotope depend on the pharmacokinetics of the isotope, itself dependent in part on the half-life of the isotope, and the pharmacodynamics of organ uptake. Information from animal experiments is used to model the expected distribution of isotope, and finally, computer modeling allows prediction of individual organ and whole body doses.

A number of radioisotopes were considered. Phosphorus-32 phosphate is a bone seeker and a balloon rupture would result in skeletal localization, and consequent bone-marrow suppression. Yttrium-90 is classified as a lanthanide element, and the Y^{3+} cation is also rapidly and effectively a bone seeker. The ramifications of marrow suppression and/or high radiation dose to other radiation-sensitive tissues in the event of the rupture of balloons containing radioactive solutions are thus major concerns with the use of yttrium-90-labeled radiopharmaceuticals. Rhenium-188, primarily a beta emitter with a maximum beta energy of 2.12 MeV, has a half-life of only 16.9 h, and is readily available by milking a $^{188}W/^{188}Re$ generator. The key, however, to the safe use of this isotope is reaction of the generator-derived ^{188}Re-perrhenate into a chemical species that is rapidly excreted in the urine.

Recently, the triglycyl peptide agent mercaptoacetylglycylglycylglycylglycine (MAG_3), exhibiting strong chelation properties for technetium-99m, has been developed[3] for imaging the renal parenchyma. Because of the availability and superior imaging characteristics of technetium-99m, Tc-99m-MAG_3 is now widely used clinically for this purpose. Rhenium is located in the same group (VIIB) as technetium in the periodic table. Since perrhenate (ReO_4^-) has chemical characteristics very similar to those of pertechnetate (TcO_4^-), the chelates prepared by the coupling of ^{188}Re-perrhenate have been developed as bifunctional chelates for the labeling of new agents for cancer therapy.[3] Because of the expected rapid urinary excretion of ^{188}Re-MAG_3 in comparison with Tc-99m-MAG_3 in conjunction with

Table 14.1 Radiation dose estimates (cGy/mCi) to humans for ^{188}Re compounds

Organ	^{188}Re-perrhenate	^{188}Re-MAG$_3$
Colon	7.3	0.017
Thyroid	4.1	0.006
Urinary bladder*	5.6	14
Total body	0.21	0.025

*Assumes spontaneous bladder evacuation every 6 h.

the commercial availability of a pharmaceutically approved 'kit', an evaluation was performed of the tissue biodistribution and urinary excretion of ^{188}Re-MAG$_3$ as a candidate for balloon inflation for coronary irradiation after PTCA.[4] Table 14.1 indicates the significant safety advantage enjoyed by ^{188}Re-MAG$_3$ compared with ^{188}Re-perrhenate.

Recently, we studied the efficacy of intravascular beta-radiation to prevent balloon injury-triggered restenosis in the porcine overstretch coronary model. Radiation was delivered by ^{188}Re liquid in a perfusion balloon, inflated for approximately 10 min, to deliver doses of as much as 25 Gy to a target point 0.5 mm into the vessel wall. Almost complete suppression of neointimal growth was noted at 30 days.[5] Previous studies have demonstrated the durability of responses to intravascular radiation for as long as 6 months.[6] Thus, animal studies suggest comparable efficacy for beta radiation delivered by this approach and gamma-radiation. Human studies will be necessary to define the utility of solution-applied beta-emitting radioisotope (SABER)-delivered radiation.

Acknowledgment

I am indebted to Drs Howard Amols, Russ Knapp, and Michael Stabin for helpful discussion, sharing of unpublished data, and continued scientific collaboration.

References

1. Teirstein P, Massullo V, Jani S et al. Catheter-based radiotherapy to inhibit restenosis after coronary stenting. *N Engl J Med* 1997; **336**(24):1697–1703.

2. Amols HI, Reinstein LE, Weinberger J. Dosimetry of a radioactive coronary balloon dilatation catheter for treatment of neointimal hyperplasia. *Med Phys* 1996; **23**(10):1783–1788.

3. Guhlke S, Diekmann D, Zamora PO et al. MAG3 p-nitrophenyl ester for Tc-99m and Re-188 labeling of amines and peptides. In: Nicolini M, Bandoli G, Mazzi U, eds. *Technetium and Rhenium in Chemistry and Nuclear Medicine*, vol 4. Padua, Italy: Editorali, 1995:363–366.

4. Knapp FF Jr, Guhlke S, Beets AL et al. Intraarterial irradiation with rhenium-188 for inhibition of restenosis after PTCA – strategy and evaluation of species for rapid urinary excretion. *J Nucl Med* 1997; **38**:124P.

5. Giedd KN, Amols H, Marboe C et al. Effectiveness of a beta-emitting liquid-filled perfusion balloon to prevent restenosis. *Circulation* 1997; **96**(8):I-220.

6. Wiedermann JG, Marboe C, Amols H et al. Intracoronary irradiation markedly reduces neointimal proliferation after balloon angioplasty in swine: persistent benefit at 6-month follow-up. *Am Coll Cardiol* 1995; **25**(6):1451–1456.

15. Isolated Liquid Beta Source Balloon Radiation Delivery System (Radiant™)

Progressive Angioplasty Systems, Menlo Park, CA, USA

Neal Eigler, James S Whiting, Raj Makkar, Ary Chernomorsky and Frank Litvack

Definition	Intravascular radiation delivery system consisting of:
	• a specialized balloon-tipped catheter filled with a liquid solution beta-radiation source
	• inflated with a shielded, pressure-regulated isotope transfer/isolation system.

History	• Multi-layer experience with solid and liquid intravascular radiation delivery systems
	• Limitations of solid and gamma systems led us to believe that a liquid uniformly distributed beta-source, centered and opposed to the arterial wall, will optimize dosimetry
	• Porcine coronary, model stent model preclinical evaluation demonstrating feasibility/safety/efficacy completed in 1997

Description (Figures 15.1–15.3)

Delivery balloon	• Over-the-wire (0.014 inch) and rapid exchange models
	• Trackable, flexible, pushable, low profile, proven PTCA and stent delivery system
	• 6 Fr compatible
	• Operating pressures < 3 atmospheres
	• Dual markers
	• Lengths 20, 30, 40 mm; diameters 2.0–4.0 mm
Isotope	Any liquid beta-source, including Re-188
Dose/target tissue	14–28 Gy at 0.5 mm depth
Exposure time	5–10 min
Operator exposure	< 5 mRem/treatment

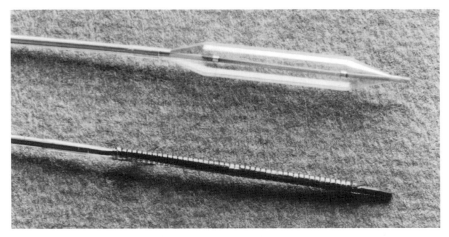

Figure 15.1 *PAS RADIANT™ isolated liquid beta source balloon. Top: Inflated dual-marker balloon. Bottom: WRAP™ balloon protective sheath to minimize profile.*

Tips and tricks

Similar to conventional balloon percutaneous transluminal coronary recanalization (PTCA). May be used before or after stent placement. The lesion should be thoroughly predilated with a fully expanded PTCA balloon of the same size intended for radiation at ≥ 6 atm prior to placing the RADIANT™ system. If the lesion has been stented, it must be fully expanded and post-dilated at ≥ 12 atm prior to placing the RADIANT™ system. The angioplaster must prepare each RADIANT™ catheter by pressurizing with air to rated burst pressure with the WRAP™ protective sheath in place. During usage, inflation with radioactive media should not exceed 3 atm.

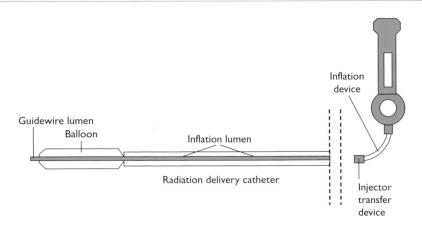

Figure 15.2 *Schematic of RADIANT™ radiation delivery system.*

Proposed indications
- Prophylaxis of de novo lesions after POBA, atherectomy, or stent
- Treatment of restenotic lesions
- Treatment of in-stent restenosis

Why we like the PAS RADIANT™

The PAS RADIANT™ uses a proven PTCA/stent delivery balloon platform. The device is easy to use and most compatible with catheterization laboratory standard operating procedures. Our isolated liquid source balloon has many advantages. It allows access to treat coronary lesions located in mid- to distal segments in tortuous vessels through ⩾ 6-Fr guiding catheters. It delivers the most homogeneous, centered, and precise dose distribution of any device. It is least affected by vagaries in vessel/lesion size or morphology. Although isotope leakage is a remote possibility, with a short half-life, and rapidly distributed and excreted radioisotope, the consequences to the patient and laboratory personnel are minimal. It is well tolerated compared with the loss or uncontrolled exposure from a long-lived solid beta or gamma source.

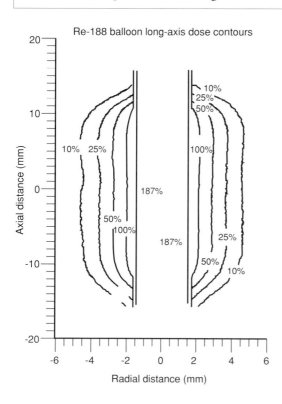

Figure 15.3 Plot of measured dose distribution of a ^{188}Re-filled balloon. Axial and radial scales differ.

Bibliography

US patents 5,302, 168 and 5,411,466.

16. THE XENACATH BRACHYTHERAPY SYSTEM

Cook Corporation, Bloomington, IN, USA

Marc G Apple and Ron Waksman

Definition A catheter-based system to deliver intracoronary xenon-133 radioactive gas into a custom shielded balloon angiography catheter. The components of the system are:

- Xenon-133 inert radiogas
- Balloon catheter, varying in size from 2.5 × 30 mm to 4.0 × 40 mm
- 'Gas-tight' syringe.

History
- **1996–1999** Benchtop dosimetry and safety studies
- **1997–1998** Primary animal coronary studies
- **1998–1999** Optimized clinical prototype design
- **1999** Initial animal peripheral vessel studies
- **2000** Pilot patient coronary trials scheduled

XenaCath description

The XenaCath balloon catheter system provides low-pressure vessel wall conformality, thereby replicating the intraluminal structure of the applied angioplasty balloon. As such, a consistent and predictable depth dose will be delivered as the xenon radiogas fills the balloon surface, allowing homogenous depth dose coverage, including deposition into the adjacent adventitia.

- The noble gas, inert properties of xenon-133 provide an excellent safety profile for practical, closed system administration, even at higher activity.
- Long-term medical use as an 'unsealed' imaging agent has demonstrated a superb safety record over several decades of administration.
- The primary emissions consist of dual production of shorter range beta particles and low-energy photons.

- The conformal xenon balloon system provides a predictable primary radiation dose profile out to 0.5–1.0 mm tissue depth, which is inherently controlled by the structure and shape of the catheter apparatus.

Advantages of xenon gas

Xenon-133 is one of the few radioisotopes of xenon (also xenon-127) with a multi-decade history of safe and routine clinical use. Typically, it has been applied in gaseous form (mixed with 95% pure carbon dioxide) or partially solubilized in saline for functional ventilation imaging or brain perfusion

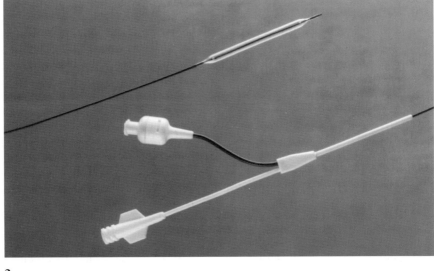

a

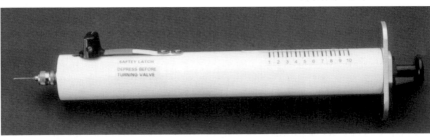

b

Figure 16.1 (a) Prototype XenaCath balloon catheter with custom scaled port assembly, unique lumen design, and integrated shielding. (b) Prototype shielded Xenon-133 'gas-tight' injector unit. Design custom fit for XenaCath catheters

imaging, as used throughout the world. Xenon-133 has a physical half-life of 5.3 days and emits both beta particles (360 kev max) and relatively low-energy gamma- and x-rays of 81 keV and 32 keV, respectively. Xenon-133 decays to a stable, non-radioactive isotope of cesium. It is produced in single unit individualized dosing ampules (Dupont) or bulk cylinders (Nordion). Therefore, because of its history of clinical use and high volume commercial radiopharmaceutical production, it is readily available, with flexible dosing and quantity as needed on a daily or weekly basis; fully dose calibrated and quality tested.

XenaCath profile

- Specialized conformal, self-centering 'gas-tight' balloon-type catheter system
- Applied over standard angioplasty guidewire; simple inflation/deflation design and control
- Multiple balloon sizes available for coronary or peripheral vessels for optimal coverage of individual lesions
- Routine treatment times of 2–5 min
- Specialized gas injector unit with customized catheter safety attachment
- Clinical benefits of inert gas and low energy emissions
- Extremely safe in vivo and environmental profile
- Predictable rapid dose rate and delivery
- Closed catheter system; average 200–300 mCi treatment
- Beta particles 360 keV peak; photons of 32 and 81 keV
- Minimal support equipment and simple external exhaust required
- Future simple 'drop and load' injector for easy individual preparation and dose delivery

---

Exposure and safety

Any free xenon-133 gas may be readily and safely exhausted from a standard directional venting system. Rapid air dilution and low-energy emissions allow for an excellent safety profile. Even in high activity concentrations or continuous low activity levels, personnel and patient dose exposure is far below safe allowances and comparatively less than most standard diagnostic procedures (see below) or other potential intravascular brachytherapy sources. Treatment time for delivered effective doses was completed, on average, in < 2.25 min; with effective dose rates of > 400–500 cGy/min.

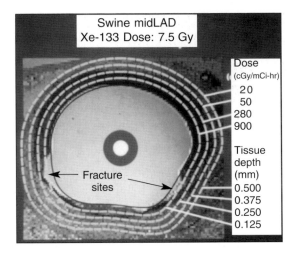

Figure 16.2 Example of actual transverse section of Xenon-133 treated swine artery. Superimposed conformal inflated balloon model to demonstrate comparative depth dosimetry at fracture site.

This system provides an all round very safe and inexpensive source which requires minimal dosimetry efforts and can administer a *consistent*, *homogeneous* prescription dose to a predictable depth, routinely.

Inventory of expensive or decay wasted radiosources can be minimized because xenon-133 could be delivered as needed for patient-variable loads and can be kept for a week.

General advantages of the XenaCath system

- Physician may remain at bedside during brachytherapy
- Expedient set-up and treatment time
- Extremely favorable radiation handling and exposure profile
- Readily available and cost-effective xenon-133 source
- Uniquely safe physical and physiological properties of inert gas
- Conformal and self-centering therapeutic dosing
- Homogeneous dose to angioplasty injury site
- Favorable dose drop-off beyond primary adventitia
- Flexibility for multiple lesions and variable sizes
- Individualized balloon size for clinical coverage
- Minimal support equipment, personnel, and related costs
- Marked, dose-dependent inhibition of restenosis in post-angioplasty porcine studies

Table 16.1 General depth dose and dose rate profile averages. Specific values are dependent on selected balloon size and composition.

Tissue depth from balloon surface (mm)	Dose rate (cGy/mCi per hour)
0.125	880–920
0.250	210–240
0.375	132–150
0.500	32–50
0.750	14–20
1.00	10–12

Summary

A xenon-133 radioactive gas catheter delivery system offers a combination of clinically effective, pragmatic, radiation exposure and cost-effective advantages—equal to or surpassing many other proposed systems. Treatment time for delivered effective doses was completed, on average, in < 2.25 min; with effective dose rates of > 400–500 cGy/min.

This system provides an all-round very safe and inexpensive source which requires minimal dosimetry efforts and can administer a consistent, homogeneous prescription dose to a predictable depth, routinely.

17. The Irradiator™

Interventional Technologies, San Diego, CA, USA

Ron Waksman

Definition and description

Local delivery of radioisotopes directly into the vessel wall by injecting the radioisotopes into the vessel via a local delivery catheter system Local drug delivery was introduced as an alternative to systemic administration of a variety of agents, which failed to reduce the restenosis rate.[1] The technology is based on the success of delivering sufficient concentration of the drug (much higher than the human body can tolerate by systemic administration) to the treated or nearby to the treated segment in the coronary tree.[2-4] The device used for this application is the Infiltrator™ (Interventional Technologies, San Diego, CA, USA). A variety of radionuclides can be injected to the vessel wall via the Infiltrator™. A vehicle to enhance delivery of the isotope will enhance the efficiency of the delivery and the residence of the isotope at the adventitia and periadventitial space.

The delivery device 'the Irradiator'

The Infiltrator™, a true intramural drug deporting system, was selected as the delivery device. This is an angioplasty balloon catheter that has three rows of small nipples on its surface (Figure 17.1). The nipples are in communication with small channels, and during inflation of the balloon the nipples penetrate into the vessel wall. The radioisotopes can be delivered through the channels of the nipples into the vessel wall and into the adventitia. The device incorporates a low-pressure positioning balloon with a series of microminiaturized injector ports mounted on its surface and connected to a fluid flow channel independent of the inflation/deflation system. The balloon has been crafted in such a way that the injector ports are recessed during maneuvering in the artery, but upon inflation these injector ports radially extend and enter the vessel wall. A multiplicity of individual ports facilitates injection of drug over an area encompassing 360' × 15 mm

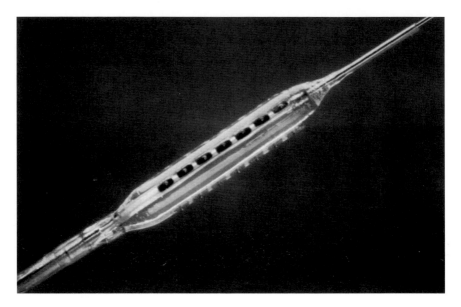

Figure 17.1 *The Infiltrator*™ *device used for delivery of* ^{99m}Tc; *note the three rows of small nipples on its surface, which are in contact with the vessel wall.*

(length). Microliter quantities of drug can therefore be delivered into the tunica media of the arterial wall in a precise fashion. Injection of the drug is accomplished in < 10 s, without substantial intimal damage and with ≥ 90% delivery efficiency and minimal luminal washout.[5,6] The coverage area can be increased with tandem applications. Including balloon up/down time, a single injection application is unlikely to take > 60 s.

Liposome encapsulation of ^{99m}Tc

It is hoped that the encapsulation of ^{99m}Tc (lipid bilayer vesicles) will improve the residence time of the isotope in the coronary artery and a rapid method for synthesis of such vesicles suitable for use in the radiopharmacy has been developed. Studies were performed using generator-produced ^{99}Tc (as $^{99m}TcO_4$), and commercially available liposome formulations of various chemistries and charges (positive, negative or neutral) to determine the efficacy and stability of encapsulation. Paper chromatography with detection by phosphor plate (Fuji) imaging and liquid scintillation was used to determine selective uptake of the isotope by the injected vessel wall (Figure 17.2). The chemistry of the neutral membrane liposome is non-toxic. The

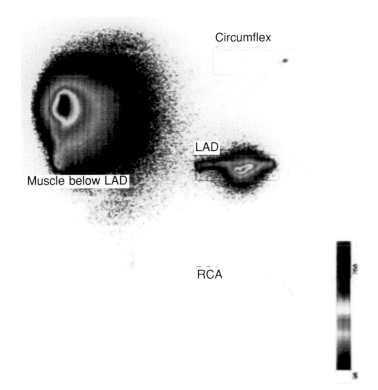

Figure 17.2 *Detection of* ^{99m}Tc *after intramural injection to the coronary artery by phosphor plate (Fuji) imaging using paper chromatography 2 h after injection. Porcine injured coronary artery (LAD) 35 min after Sestamibi (2.5 mCi) application with injury.*

encapsulation efficiency of ^{99m}Tc was consistently of the order of 97% for all chemistries and there was no measurable leakage of ^{99m}Tc from the liposomes during the time course followed.

This approach demonstrates the rapidity by which ^{99m}Tc can be packaged for delivery to the perfusion site after PTCA. The fact that liposome-encapsulated ^{99m}Tc resides at the perfusion site with less washout than free ^{99}Tc suggests the possibility of using this same method for other isotopes.

Isotopes proposed for this technology

- 99-Technetium
- Seastamibi
- Ceretec

141

History and preclinical investigation

- Prior studies with this device have demonstrated that small amounts of fluid (0.4 ml) can be delivered into the vessel wall without acute or significant subacute damage to the wall and without escape of the substance.
- Injection of the drug is accomplished in < 10 s, without substantial intimal damage and with ≥ 90% delivery efficiency and minimal luminal washout.[5,6]
- Clinical trial using the Infiltrator™ for intracoronary drug delivery.[7]
- The ability to deliver free ^{99}Tc versus encapsulated ^{99}Tc in liposomes directly into the arterial wall of 12 porcine coronaries was examined by injecting 0.4 ml of the isotopes (4–14 mCi) via the IABC.
- Studies proved the principle that radionuclides can be delivered safely locally to the vessel wall. Liposome-^{99m}Tc resides longer in the vessel wall compared with free ^{99}Tc.[8]
- Liposome-^{99m}Tc was activities between 4 and 14 mCi injected following balloon injury into the vessel wall. At 4 weeks following the treatment the animals were killed and histomorphometric studies were performed. Safety was demonstrated reduction of neointima awaiting dose–response study.[9]

Advantages of the system

- Allows immediate delivery of the isotopes to the vessel before or after injury.
- Provides centering in the vessel.
- Proximity of the isotope to the target area.
- Use of radionuclides available for nuclear imaging.
- Simple to operate and to administer.
- Fast administration, <1 min for delivery of the radionuclides to the vessel wall.

Future directions

- The challenge of this technology is to be able to deliver cumulative doses of 10–15 Gy locally into the adventitia. These doses, based on the catheter-based systems, should be sufficient to reduce the intimal hyperplasia following balloon injury.
- Further isotopes such as Ceretec are being tested to obtain significant reduction of the neointima formation following injury in the porcine model.
- Clinical trials will take place once the appropriate isotope and the dose have been determined.

References

1. Wolinsky H, Taubman MD. Local delivery to the arterial wall: pharmacologic and molecular approaches. In: Holmes DR Jr, Vlietstra RE, eds. *Coronary Balloon Angioplasty*. Boston: Blackwell, 1994:156–186.

2. Riessen R, Isner JM. Prospects for site-specific delivery of pharmacologic and molecular therapies. *J Am Coll Cardiol* 1994; **23**:1234–1244.

3. Fernando-Ortiz A, Meyer BJ, Mailhac A et al. A new approach for local intravascular drug delivery: iontophoretic balloon. *Circulation* 1994; **89**:1518–1522.

4. Rogers C, Karnovsky MJ, Edelman ER. Inhibition of experimental neointimal hyperplasia and thrombosis depends on type of vascular injury and the site of drug administration. *Circulation* 1993; **88**:1215–1221.

5. Wiedermann JG, Marboe C, Schwartz A, Amols H, Weinberger J. Intracoronary irradiation reduces restenosis after balloon angioplasty in a porcine model. *J Am Coll Cardiol* 1994; **23**:1491–1498.

6. Barath P, Popov A, Dillehay GL, Matos G, McKiernan T. Infiltrator angioplasty balloon catheter: a device for combined angioplasty and intramural site-specific treatment. *Cathet Cardiovasc Diagn* 1997; **41**:333–341.

7. Pavlides GS, Barath P, Maginas A, Vasilikos V, Cokkinos DV, ONeill WW. Intramural drug delivery by direct injection within the arterial wall: first clinical experience with a novel intracoronary delivery-infiltrator system. *Cathet Cardiovasc Diagn* 1997; **41**:287–292.

8. Karam LR, Zimmerman BE, Chan RC, Waksman R. Liposome encapsulation of ^{99m}Tc for use in intravascular brachytherapy. *Adv Cardiovasc Radiat Ther* 1998; Syllabus 33 (abstract 29).

9. Waksman R, Chan RC, Kim WH et al. Injection of radionuclides to the coronary arterial wall: Hot arteries: a novel vascular brachytherapy approach to reduce restenosis. *Circulation* 1998; **98**:I-652:3425.

18. RDX™ Radiation Delivery System: Balloon-based Radiation Therapy

Novoste Corporation, Norcross, CA, USA

Maurice Buchbinder, Gary Strathearn, Lisa A Tam and Brett Trauthen

Background

Intravascular brachytherapy has become a promising technique for the treatment of restenosis. Several studies have reported reductions in the restenosis rates to as low as 10–15%, even in lesion types prone to recurrence.[1–4] Animal investigations into the mechanism of this therapy have shown that ionizing radiation inhibits the formation of neointimal tissue in response to the injury following balloon angioplasty.[5]

The first studies of intracoronary brachytherapy adapted Ir-192 ribbons from radiation oncology for use in coronary arteries. The use of this high-energy gamma source presents several challenges to the physician, however. Depending on the activity of the source, protecting laboratory personnel from radiation requires over a centimeter of lead to effectively block the emissions while the source is in the patient. Hence, most studies utilizing this isotope require that the laboratory staff vacate the room during the radiation treatment, which can last over 15 min.

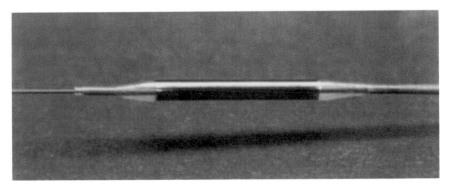

Figure 18.1 Radiance balloon catheter.

To address these issues, several new systems have been proposed that utilize high-energy beta-emitting isotopes such as Sr/Y-90, P-32, and Re-188.[6] Beta sources such as these can be shielded with plastics instead of lead, but the limited penetration depth of beta particles through the tissue makes these sources very sensitive to position within the vessel, making source centering an important consideration for treatment, especially in larger vessels. Moreover, all of the systems proposed to date require calibration and the aid of a medical physicist for dosimetry calculations.

RDX technology

In a novel approach to intracoronary brachytherapy, the RDX radiation delivery system (Radiance Medical Systems, Irvine, CA, USA), seeks to overcome the disadvantages of beta isotopes through a new source and delivery system design. Designed specifically for use in the cardiac catheterization laboratory, the RDX incorporates the P-32 isotope directly into the balloon material of a PTCA-type catheter, as shown in Figure 18.1. This approach takes advantage of source apposition to the vessel wall, thereby simultaneously exploiting the beta characteristic of a short penetration depth and eliminating the need for centering. In addition, direct vessel apposition of the source reduces the required activity to deliver therapeutic doses to the target tissue, allowing simplistic shielding and a disposable device design. The disposable aspect eliminates the need for constant source re-calibration and dosimetry calculation before each usage. Generally, the RDX system is a simple device to deliver since it utilizes the same delivery techniques as standard angioplasty.

The first consideration for any brachytherapy system is the choice of isotope. Given the advantages and limitations of both the gamma and beta isotopes mentioned earlier, the optimum source design is the use of a beta isotope characterized by a delivery system design providing proximity to the target tissue and concentricity with respect to the target tissue.

Generally speaking, particle energy, whether beta or gamma, dictates its suitability for use in brachytherapy. Experiments and dosimetry models suggest that gamma emitters must have a minimum average emission energy of 20–30 keV, while beta emitters must have a minimum average energy of about 700 keV[7,8] to achieve adequate penetration into the vessel wall. A second important criterion for usage of a given isotope is its half-life. Although a longer half-life is desirable for a reusable source, a disposable device requires a shorter half-life in order to decrease the decay time before disposal. A 2–3 week shelf-life is reasonable for a disposable system considering the waste management issues.

146

Several isotopes meeting these criteria were considered for use in the RDX, most notably I-125 and Pd-103 among gamma isotopes, and P-32, Sr/Y-90 and W/Re-188 among beta isotopes. Of these, I-125 and Sr/Y-90 activities were deemed too hazardous for a disposable system. W/Re-188 and Pd-103 were not readily available in a high specific activity. Given the requirements, P-32 appeared to be the best overall choice of isotope. Its half-life is close to ideal for a disposable product, and it is commonly available at high specific activities (> 150 00 μCi/μg).

Once the choice of isotope was determined, a completely new source technology was developed specifically for the RDX. The source was constructed using a proprietary 'attachment' system that binds the isotope onto a substrate through a chemical reaction. This attachment technique can be performed on almost any surface. In the case of the RDX, a thin plastic film was chosen as the substrate in order to minimize the balloon profile. In this particular case, sheets are customized and cut in length and width to match the final balloon size. The source sheets are then wrapped around the RDX catheter balloon, and sealed within a secondary cover, forming a tri-layer system. Generally, the greatest concern for any thin film solid source had been the ability to attach enough activity to enable the delivery of an adequate dose with a maximum treatment time of 10 min. In the case of the RDX, which uses P-32, < 1 μg of isotope is required to achieve the necessary dose-rate to the target tissue.

The delivery system design for the RDX is similar to that of a conventional balloon angioplasty catheter. It is a 0.014-inch wire compatible device constructed in over-the-wire or rapid-exchange configuration. Its profile and flexibility are similar to a stent delivery system. As mentioned earlier, the balloon itself has a unique tri-layer construction as shown in Figure 18.2. The encapsulation of the radiation source within the balloon layers seals it from

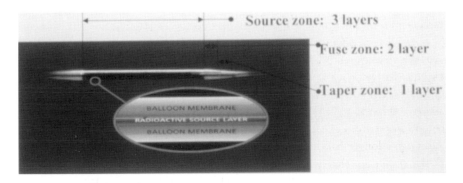

Figure 18.2 Tri-layer construction of the balloon.

direct contact with both the blood stream and the inflation fluid. The balloon membranes are constructed from a mixture of materials specifically designed for this purpose.

To date, the RDX system has undergone aggressive in vitro and in vivo testing. The balloon is designed to fully inflate at 2 atmospheres (atm) of pressure. This low operating pressure was intentionally chosen to minimize the potential for barotrauma to the vessel wall. The integrity of the source seal under cyclic conditions appears to be excellent. In qualification tests, each balloon underwent 120 inflation cycles at 1 atm above the operating pressure without damaging the balloon or compromising the source. The behavior of the RDX under balloon burst conditions is an important design consideration. Using different compositions and dimensions for each layer of the balloon, the relative strength of each zone within the balloon can be varied (see Figure 18.2). By making the single-layer 'taper zone' the weakest, the failure mode of the balloon can be directed to this area. When the balloon breaks here, the source is not compromised and only contrast media escapes into the bloodstream.

Performance

Dosimetry models and direct measurements have been undertaken at several laboratories, including the National Institute of Science and Technology (NIST) in Washington, DC and Cedars-Sinai Medical Center in Los Angeles. The results of these studies showed remarkable dose-rate efficiency of the RDX source (Gy/mCi per min) compared with other source configurations using the same isotope. This result is due to the enhanced proximity of the source relative to the target tissue. Figure 18.3 compares the dose rate vs depth in tissue for different ^{32}P sources (P-32 wire, P-32 liquid-filled balloons, and the RDX P-32 balloon). As can be seen in this model, the RDX system dose-rate is three to four times higher than the other configurations. As a result, the RDX source requires three to four times less activity to deliver a similar dose rate. For example, if one desires a prescription dose of 20 Gy given to a depth of 1 mm in 5 min to a 25-mm long lesion, a 0.5-mm wire source requires approximately 100 mCi of P-32, a liquid isotope filled balloon requires 75 mCi, and the RDX source requires only 30 mCi. This reduction in activity translates to a lessened exposure risk for the patient and laboratory personnel.

The dosimetry characteristics of the RDX were made using two different types of phantoms. As can be seen in Figure 18.4, both axial and linear images of the source were taken and analysed. In all cases, calibrated

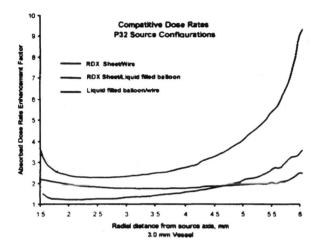

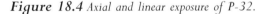

Figure 18.3 *Comparison dose rate vs depth in tissue for different P-32 sources (P-32 wire; P-32 liquid-filled balloons, and the RDX P-32 balloon).*

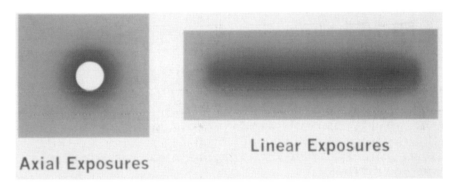

Figure 18.4 *Axial and linear exposure of P-32.*

GAFchromic™ film was used to record dose measurements. These images show the uniform penetration of the radiation around the surface of the balloon, and the uniformity of the radiation along the source surface.

Stenting is expected to be a common adjunctive procedure to radiation, so the effect of the stent on the dose was studied. The apposition of the RDX source to the vessel wall appears to greatly reduce the impact of metal shielding. This rather unique property is illustrated in Figure 18.5, which shows a dosimetric image of the RDX within a stent in both a deflated and an inflated, or deployed, condition. As can be seen, the stent strut pattern is readily apparent owing to the shielding effect (shadowing) of the metal strut on the beta particles in the deflated condition. In the inflated condition, the

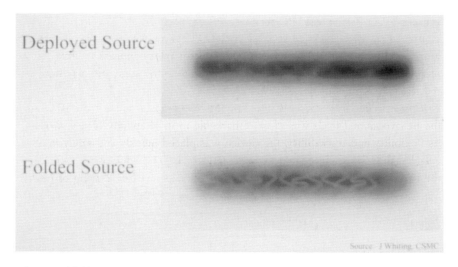

Figure 18.5 *Dosimetric image of the RDX within a stent in both a deflated and an inflated, or deployed, condition.*

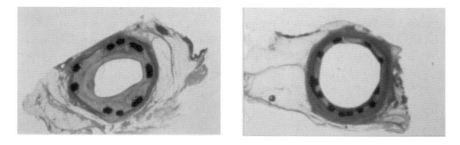

Figure 18.6 *Control (left) versus irradiator following stent implantation 18 Gy at 1-mm depth (RDX system).*

image of the stent is difficult to discern. The proximity of the source to the stent reduces the shielding effect of the stent on the delivery of radiation. This particular study verifies the concern that stents can indeed block some of the beta particles and hence affect the uniformity of the dose. This is especially applicable to beta sources that are not in close proximity to the stent. In this study, metallic stents appear to reduce the overall dose-rate to the surrounding tissue by < 10–12%.

In preparation for clinical studies, the RDX system has been tested in over 40 animals. Using a classical porcine stent-injury model, the RDX system has been used to administer doses ranging from 10 to 40 Gy at a 1-mm depth. At 1 month, there is a significant reduction in neointimal formation within the treated segments compared with control vessels at doses over 15 Gy. These findings are consistent with similar reported studies using wire and seed sources.[9,10] An example of the radiation effect using the RDX is shown in Figure 18.6, where a dose of 18 Gy at a 1-mm depth was delivered, showing unremarkable neointimal formation. The control artery appears to have marked neointimal growth completely surrounding the stent and significantly reducing the lumen of the vessel.

These results are extremely encouraging. The performance of the RDX in the in vivo animal trials was most remarkable in its simplicity of use. Given its flexibility and trackability, the device was placed quickly and safely in all vessels. Although slightly larger than a standard balloon angioplasty catheter, the tip profile of the RDX remains very good, allowing for crossing of freshly implanted stents, even in small vessels.

Clinical studies

The first human trial of the RDX system is scheduled for late summer 1999 as part of an international multi-center feasibility study involving approximately 150 patients. In an open-label prospective registry, named the 'BETTER' study (BEta radiation Trial To Eliminate Restenosis), the RDX will be evaluated in both de novo and restenotic lesions (stented and non-stented). Concurrently, the RDX will undergo evaluation in a randomized clinical trial testing its safety and efficacy for in-stent restenosis named the BRITE study (Beta Radiation to reduce In-stent resTEnosis).

Summary

The RDX system represents an exciting new generation of radiation-delivering systems. The system design is primarily aimed at simplifying intracoronary brachytherapy in the catheterization laboratory setting. Utilizing the concept of 'proximity' between radiation source and target tissue, the RDX uses as little isotope as possible with uniform dosimetry, even in the presence of obstacles such as a stent.

In the course of developing this concept, an entirely novel radiation source technology was invented. Theoretical dosimetry models predicted an increase in dose delivery efficiency that has since been proven by quantitative studies showing superior treatment characteristics. The promise of the RDX was validated in animal investigations because this system achieved a similar degree of neointimal inhibition to that reported with other radioactive systems. Clinical studies are due to begin in the near future, and expectations for this system remain very high.

References

1. Tierstein P, et al. Catheter-based radiotherapy to inhibit restenosis after coronary stenting. *N Engl J Med* 1997; **336**:1697–1703.

2. King SB III, et al. Endovascular β-radiation to reduce restenosis after coronary balloon angioplasty – results of the Beta Energy Restenosis Trial (BERT). *Circulation* 1998; **97**:2025–2030.

3. Verin Y, et al. Feasibility of intracoronary β-irradiation to reduce restenosis after balloon angioplasty. *Circulation* 1997; **95**:1138–1144.

4. Condado J, et al. Long-term angiographic and clinical outcome after percutaneous transluminal coronary angioplasty and intracoronary radiation therapy in humans. *Circulation* 1997; **96**:728–732.

5. Waksman R, et al. Intracoronary low-dose β-irradiation inhibits neointima formation after coronary artery balloon injury in the swine restenosis model. *Circulation* 1995; **92**:3025–3031.

6. Waksman R, et al. *Handbook of Vascular Brachytherapy*. London: Martin Dunitz, 1998.

7. Amols H. Review of endovascular brachytherapy physics for prevention of restenosis. *Cardiovascular Radiation Medicine* 1999; **1**:64–71.

8. Nath R, et al. On the depth of penetration of photons and electrons for intravascular brachytherapy. *Cardiovascular Radiation Medicine* 1999; **1**:72–79.

9. Wiedermann JG, et al. Intracoronary irradiation markedly reduces restenosis after balloon angioplasty in a porcine model. *J Am Coll Cardiol* 1994; **23**:1491–1498.

10. Waksman R, et al. Intracoronary radiation before stent implantation inhibits neointima formation in stented porcine coronary arteries. *Circulation* 1995; **92**:1383–1386.

19. BRACHYTHERAPY GUIDED BY ULTRASOUND

Department of Radiation Oncology, Cleveland Clinic Foundation, Cleveland, OH, USA

Jay P Ciezki

Introduction

Intravascular brachytherapy as a prophylaxis for restenosis after transcatheter vascular intervention is very promising.[1-3] Clearly, we are in the introductory phase of an exciting new therapy. The initial trials are now being completed and although the results point to intravascular brachytherapy as a highly efficacious treatment, failure analyses are demonstrating directions that may be taken for optimization. The use of intravascular ultrasound (IVUS) as a guide during the delivery of intravascular brachytherapy may provide the desired improvements.

Why IVUS? Recently, medical device manufacturers have either closed down or limited their IVUS product lines. Third-party payers reimburse poorly for its use. Obviously, the value of IVUS in its current form and application is being questioned from several perspectives. This may be because current transcatheter vascular intervention technology either does not allow the clinician to respond to the vascular imaging supplied by IVUS or there is scant evidence that such responses have clinical benefit. Most transcatheter vascular intervention is a response to angiographic or luminal anatomy. It cannot react to vascular wall imaging any more elegantly than changing its radial force/size or the number of times it is deployed. The vascular wall matters little, except in settings like dissection, to the acute results of the therapy, so vascular wall image guidance would not be expected to improve these existing methods of vascular intervention.

Intravascular brachytherapy, and brachytherapy in general, differs in that it is a highly geographically specific therapy that may be greatly enhanced by ultrasound guidance. A good parallel may be drawn with prostate brachytherapy. The efficacy and safety of transperineal prostate implantation has been improved with the use of transrectal ultrasound guidance to adequately cover the treatment target and minimize the irradiation of surrounding structures.[4,5] A similar optimization should occur with intravascular brachytherapy as the treatment targets are identified. Work in human tissue bank arterial sections that received percutaneous transluminal coronary angioplasty (PTCA) prior to death demonstrates the ubiquitous nature of cell proliferation (a reasonable target for intravascular brachytherapy) after PTCA in humans. In this study, proliferating cell nuclear antigen (PCNA) was used to detect proliferating cells in the arterial wall. There was no correlation between cell proliferation and the arterial region (plaque, plaque shoulder, or region with lowest plaque burden), arterial layer (intima, media, adventitia), or evidence of a prior intervention.[6] The failure analysis from the Scripps Trial also helps identification of the target tissue. In attempting to correlate success with several radiotherapeutic and clinical variables, a pronounced effect was found in favor of success by achieving a dose of at least 8 Gy to the adventitial border (and therefore the proliferating cells it contains) as seen on IVUS ($P = 0.009$).[7] Mindful of this information, it seems reasonable to target the entire vessel wall for irradiation to a dose of at least 8 Gy. The remainder of this chapter will discuss how this may be done safely.

Design rationale and device description

The apparent importance of the vascular wall anatomy to the success of intravascular brachytherapy means that a device should allow the clinician to make the radiation conform to the wall's peculiarities. Although each lesion is unique, one theme common to the axial anatomy is the eccentric nature of the plaque, as well as the eccentric dwell position of a catheter that has been placed across the lesion.[8] The relationship between axial anatomy and a typical radiation dose profile may be seen in Figure 19.1. This figure depicts one method of optimization: centering the radioactive source in the lumen. Notice the range of dose to the adventitia ($\sim$ 6 Gy at the far side and $\sim$ 20 Gy to the near side). With this arrangement, the dose to the far side can only be increased by increasing the dwell time of the source. The price paid for this is the possibility of excessive dose to the near vessel wall. The consequences of this may be seen in some preclinical and clinical studies. Histology from an animal study shows focal vessel wall necrosis that is likely to be the result of excessive radiation dose where the radiation source was lying against the vessel wall.[9] Angiography from the human study demonstrates a possible long-term result of focal vessel wall necrosis: ectasia of the treated segment.[10] Prolonged dwell time of a radioactive source does not appear to be an entirely satisfactory answer.

The approach taken with the present device is to utilize dose profile modification to match the anatomy. In other words, eccentric dose profiles for

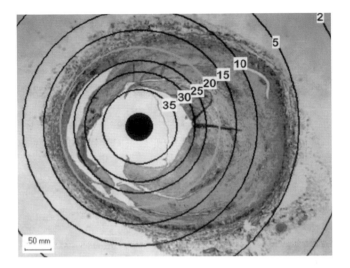

Figure 19.1 *An example of a tissue section from a patient who received PTCA 1 day prior to death with the dose profile of a* ^{188}*Re source superimposed. The concentric circles emanating from the source (black dot centered in lumen) represent the dose in Gray (Gy). Note that the far side of the adventitia receives about 6 Gy when 20 Gy is prescribed at 1.5 mm.*

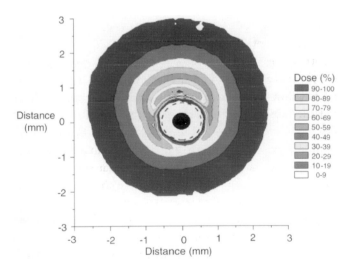

Figure 19.2 *The radiation dose profile modification that can be achieved with attenuators imbedded in the catheter wall on the same* ^{188}*Re source. Notice that the design forces a more intense, and therefore penetrating, area from the 10 to 1 o'clock positions. Also note that the dark band (the 19–10% isodose area) remains unaltered around the entire circumference. Within this relatively broad area the dose varies by ~ 10% of maximum. This enhances the homogeneity of dose delivery because it permits the vessel to move substantially within its bounds with very little dose variation.*

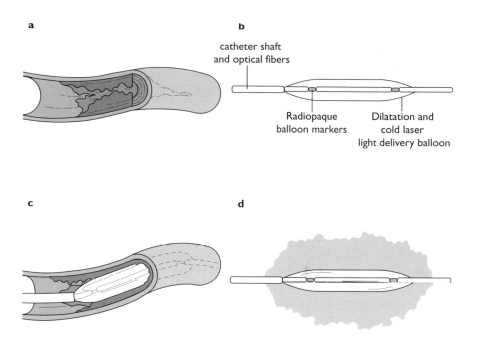

a

b

catheter shaft
and optical fibers

Radiopaque
balloon markers

Dilatation and
cold laser
light delivery balloon

c

d

Figure 19.3 *An overlay of the arterial section from Figure 19.1 and the dose profile from Figure 19.2. Note that the adventitia remains within the 19–10% isodose area.*

eccentric anatomy. This is done by modifying the intensity of the radiation at various positions around the source's circumference. The effect on the dose profile can be seen in Figure 19.2. The partial attenuation of the dose profile forms an eccentric distribution of dose. It forces a more intense and penetrating area of dose in the 10 to 1 o'clock positions in Figure 19.2, while moderating the area of dose in the remainder of the dose distribution in Figure 19.2. One may imagine an orientation of this system in an artery where the penetrating areas of dose are aimed at the far vessel wall (very likely through a plaque) and the moderately dosed areas are adjacent to the near vessel wall. Figure 19.3 demonstrates this arrangement. The net result is a homogenization of dose to the target vessel wall, enabling the clinician to stay within any therapeutic window with greater ease.

The attainment of the dose homogenization described above requires three things working in concert: dose profile modification, vascular wall imaging, and the ability to change the catheter's axial orientation in response to the anatomy. Dose profile modification is achieved by imbedding radiation attenuators in the catheter wall. IVUS provides the necessary vascular wall imaging. Solid-state IVUS gives superior imaging because of its low image

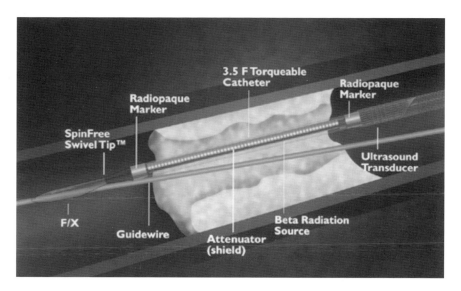

Figure 19.4 *An illustration of the catheter in situ. The catheter's guidewire lumen is contained in a segment that allows free rotation of it relative to the rest of the catheter. This prevents guidewire prolapse and entanglement during torquing.*

distortion as compared with mechanical systems.[11] In addition, it allows fiducial markers representing the orientation of the dose profile to be projected over the image of the vascular wall. The ability to respond to the anatomy depicted by IVUS is achieved by physically linking the attenuator-containing catheter segment immediately adjacent to the IVUS transducer in a known position, and mounting the conglomeration on a shaft that transmits torque well. This device combines all three elements in an integrated fashion as seen in Figure 19.4.

Method of use

This catheter is passed across a lesion over a 0.014-inch guidewire; since it contains an integrated IVUS transducer, it is useful as a diagnostic and therapeutic device. The clinician may use the catheter to perform any standard diagnostic work-up thought necessary before using it for brachytherapy. The use of the catheter for radiation purposes is stepwise and methodical.

The first step is to pass the catheter across the lesion and survey it. The clinician should be looking for the axial section that represents the most dosimetrically challenging section. 'Most dosimetrically challenging' is defined

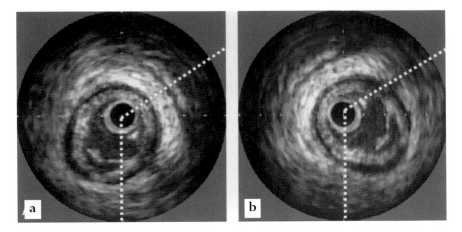

Figure 19.5 (a) An IVUS of a treatment segment prior to proper axial positioning. The dashed lines emanating from the center describe the attenuator's location. The section from 2 to 6 o'clock is the unattenuated area. In this image the catheter is not properly oriented. The unattenuated section should be aimed at the far vessel wall (the area with the dissection). (b) The same axial section after torquing into proper orientation. Now the more penetrating, unattenuated section is aimed at the far vessel wall. This would be a good image to use for dose prescription calculations.

as the most eccentric catheter placement relative to the adventitia. The length of artery to be surveyed is the length of the radiation segment of the catheter. For the sake of demonstration, this length will be taken as 15 mm.

The second step is to orient the catheter in the artery so as to achieve the most homogeneous dose to the adventitia. Invariably, this is a position in which the high intensity portion of the dose distribution is directed towards the adventitia that is furthest from the catheter. Very often, it is the adventitia behind the area of greatest plaque burden. Torquing the catheter until the IVUS image indicates that the dose profile is in the aforementioned orientation delivers the desired dose homogenization. Figure 19.5 demonstrates the procedure. From this image (Figure 19.5b), the radiation oncologist and medical physicist can calculate the dwell time of the radiation source to give the appropriate dose. The easiest way to do this is to prescribe a dose to a point on the adventitia behind the attenuated portion that the user does not wish to exceed, such as 30 Gy. If this were done with the [188]Re source from Figure 19.2 in the artery from Figure 19.5, the far side of the adventitia would receive ~ 16 Gy.

The third step is a pullback of the device into proper longitudinal position. This is done while maintaining the axial position achieved during step two. Because this catheter is made to transmit torque, it also resists torque, so the previously achieved axial position is easily maintained during pullback (the feasibility testing phase did not disclose any incidents of misalignment during pullback). If, during pullback, the catheter torques out of position, the operator will notice this by visual feedback as the IVUS image spins and by tactile feedback as the catheter spins. Should this happen, step two should be repeated. The 'proper longitudinal position' is one in which the radiation segment subtends the arterial segment to be treated. The radiation segment is easily identified on fluoroscopy because of its radiopacity. In this instance it would be 15 mm long and mounted immediately distal to the IVUS transducer.

Step four is the afterloading of the catheter with the radioactive source. The radiation oncologist pushes the source through the catheter lumen and observes the fluoroscope as the source enters the radiation segment. This is easily seen because the source and the radiation segment are radiopaque. Once the source reaches its position the dwell time starts. The source is retracted at the end of the dwell time.

One tremendous advantage of this system is that it allows for segmental radiation with a great margin of safety. Given that each lesion varies not only in axial dimensions, but also in longitudinal dimensions, the need to treat a variety of lesion lengths becomes clear. It is also clear that to use a very long source and prescribe to a set distance from the source will result in tremendous dose inhomogeneity because of the taper of the vessel's caliber. The distal portion will receive a greater dose than the proximal portion because of its proximity to the catheter. Segmenting any given length will allow prescription at distances suitable to its axial dimensions and almost customizing the brachytherapy procedure. The segments can be abutted with the help of fluoroscopy and IVUS to insure adequate, but not excessive, dosing to the entire length.

Theoretical limitations and preclinical testing

The previously described design and method of use appears elegant when considering a single axial IVUS or histological image, but what about a real vessel with a third dimension, particularly one with a tortuous lumen? The expectation is that the device will treat a single section homogeneously and treat the remainder of the length heterogeneously. In fact, careful consideration of the radiation dose profile in Figure 19.2 and the effects of segmentation of the target vessel segment, reveals that this is unlikely to happen.

First, the eccentrically modified dose profile will be considered. A review of Figure 19.2 will demonstrate two major features that enhance its ease of use. One feature is the fact that the intense area of dose is confined to an area

159

that makes up about 17% of the entire circumference. This may lead to overdosing an area of vessel wall, but this occurs only if there is a 180° change in the position of the catheter relative to the vessel wall. In a treatment segment length of 15 mm this would be hemodynamically unstable and highly unlikely. The other feature is the maintenance of the plateau phase of the dose fall off around the entire circumference of the catheter. In Figure 19.2, broad (~ 1 mm) bands of color can be seen, indicating that there is relatively little change in dose with distance in this area. The advantage to this is that the catheter can move by up to 1.5 mm relative to the vessel wall and the dose to the target will still stay within a therapeutic window of 8–30 Gy if the prescription guidelines furnished in the previous section are followed.

Second, the effects of segmentation of the treatment segment will be considered. As stated earlier, vessel tortuosity is almost always present; however, hemodynamic factors limit the degree to which it can exist. If severe tortuosity occurs over a short segment of vessel, turbulent flow occurs and this is generally not sustainable over the long term. However, severe tortuosity can occur in a chronic sense over long (> 15 mm) segments of vessel and still maintain laminar flow. Obviously, the day-to-day use of this device will require confrontation of this scenario. Segmentation of the treatment segment into lengths that are unlikely to be affected by severe tortuosity is a simple answer. A treatment segment of 15 mm will nearly ensure that the negative effects of heterogeneous radiation dosing discussed earlier will not be seen.

Confident of the advantages of this system, we have been performing preclinical animal studies with the device. In an attempt to overquantify the potential problems with the device, we used a catheter with a treatment segment of 25 mm so that vessel tortuosity issues would result in a higher likelihood of overdosing the target. We followed the prescription guidelines from the previous section on porcine coronaries that received a balloon overexpansion injury with a balloon sized to ~ 1.3–1.5 of the vessel diameter. The results of the acute cohort of animals demonstrated no evidence of vessel wall necrosis as might be expected if the vessel wall received an excessive dose. A series of animals will also be sacrificed at 6 months to ascertain the long-term effects of the device, with clinical trials soon to follow.

Summary

The present device grew out of a need to deliver radiation dose homogeneously to a vessel after transcatheter vascular intervention. This need was identified through a review of preclinical and clinical failure analyses that hint at a therapeutic window to respect. This approach builds on the successful track record of other image-guided brachytherapy procedures that have enhanced efficacy and decreased toxicity as they have become more attuned to the biology and anatomy of their target sites. This device should be poised to be a success in the emerging field of intravascular brachytherapy.

References

1. Teirstein P, Massullo V, Jani S et al. Catheter-based radiotherapy to inhibit restenosis after coronary stenting. *N Engl J Med* 1997; **336**:1697–1703.

2. Schopohl B, Liermann D, Pohlit LJ et al. Ir-192 endovascular brachytherapy for avoidance of intimal hyperplasia after percutaneous transluminal angioplasty and stent implantation in peripheral vessels: 6 years of experience. *Int J Radiat Oncol Biol Phys* 1996; **36**:835–840.

3. King III SB, Williams DO, Chougule P et al. Endovascular β-radiation to reduce restenosis after coronary balloon angioplasty results of the beta energy restenosis trial (BERT). *Circulation* 1998; **97**:2025–2030.

4. Wallner K. An improved method for computerized tomography-planned transperineal iodine 125 prostate implants. *Oncology* 1991; **5**:115–122.

5. Ragde H, Elgamal AA, Snow P et al. Ten-year disease free survival after transperineal sonography-guided iodine-125 brachytherapy with or without 45-gray external beam irradiation in the treatment of patients with clinically localized, low to high Gleason grade prostate carcinoma. *Cancer* 1998; **83**:989–1001.

6. Ciezki J, Hafeli U, Song P et al. Parenchymal cell proliferation in coronary arteries after percutaneous transluminal coronary angioplasty: a human tissue bank study. *Int J Radiat Oncol Biol Phys* 1999; **45**:963–968.

7. Teirstein P, Massullo V, Jani S et al. A subgroup analysis of the Scripps coronary radiation to inhibit proliferation poststenting trial. *Int J Radiat Oncol Biol Phys* 1998; **42**:1097–1104.

8. Berglund H, Luo H, Nishioka T et al. Highly localized arterial remodeling in patients with coronary atherosclerosis. *Circulation* 1997; **96**:1470–1476.

9. Mazur W, Ali Islam Khan, Ali M et al. High dose rate intracoronary radiation for inhibition of neointimal formation in the stented and balloon-injured porcine models of restenosis: angiographic, morphometric, and histopathologic analysis. *Int J Radiat Oncol Biol Phys* 1996; **36**:777–788.

10. Condado J, Waksman R, Gurdiel O et al. Long-term angiographic and clinical outcome after percutaneous transluminal coronary angioplasty and intracoronary radiation in humans. *Circulation* 1997; **96**:727–732.

161

11. Kimura B, Bhargava V, Palinski W, Russo R, DeMaria A. Distortion of intravascular ultrasound images because of nonuniform angular velocity of mechanical-type transducers. *Am Heart J* 1996; **132**:328–336.

20. THE SOFT X-RAY SYSTEM

XRT Corp., St Paul, MN, USA

Victor I Chornenky

Description	An intravascular catheter for local delivery of x-ray radiation to the site of angioplasty. It comprises a miniature x-ray emitter connected to the distal end of a coaxial cable placed into a delivery sheath (Figure 20.1). Once the catheter is positioned and activated, the x-ray emitter is automatically pulled back along the lesion, delivering a preprogrammed dose profile along the vessel. To cool the emitter, saline flush is provided inside the delivery sheath.

History	• **1997** New device: proof of principle is demonstrated
	• **1999** The first prototype of intravascular catheter developed
	• **1999** Animal trials
	• **2000** Clinical trials

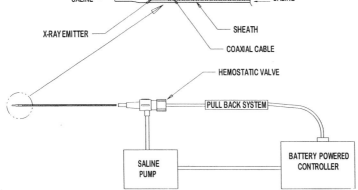

Figure 20.1 *The soft x-ray system. Schematic representation of the soft x-ray system, currently under development at XRT Corp. The x-ray emitter, shown at the distal end of a coaxial cable, comprises an anode and a cold cathode mounted in a miniature vacuum tube. The vacuum tube is made of a high dielectric strength insulator. To activate the system DC voltage (20 kV) is applied to the tube. Electrons emitted by the cold cathode are accelerated by the electrical field and impinge on the anode, emitting x-ray radiation.*

A conductive coating is deposited on the external surface of the vacuum tube. It completes the electric circuit of the emitter and provides filtration of the lower energy x-ray radiation, thereby increasing penetration ability of the radiation.

The penetration ability of X-ray radiation is characterized by the half-value layer (HVL), the thickness of a medium at which intensity of the radiation drops by half (Figure 20.2). For successful therapeutic irradiation of a given target, the HVL must have an adequate value. In the case of intravascular irradiation it should be high enough to deliver a therapeutic dose to the adventitia, but low enough to spare the myocardium and pericardium. It should also be safe for the operator and catheterization laboratory staff. Keeping in mind the size of both coronary and peripheral vessels, the adequate HVL falls between 2 and 10 mm. The lower value approximately matches the penetration ability of a ^{90}Y radioactive beta source and, probably, is the lowest practically acceptable value. Unlike beta and gamma radiation, the tissue penetration of x-rays does not depend on the properties of nuclei, and can be tailored by an adequate selection of two parameters of design: operating voltage and filtration. For operating voltages in the range of 20–25 kV in combination with appropriate filtration, a HVL of 4–10 mm, correspondingly, can be achieved easily.

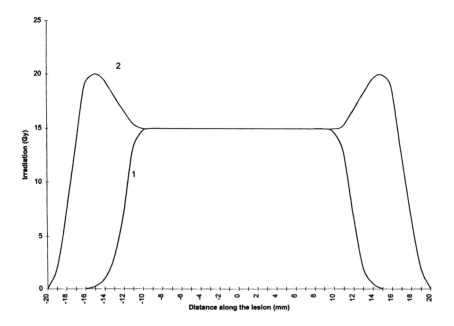

Figure 20.2 Irradiation patterns of the x-ray catheter.

The x-ray emitter consumes 1 W power. To cool the emitter, a continuous saline solution is pumped through the sheath. Computer simulations and experimental measurements indicate that a saline flow rate of 10–15 ml/min is adequate to keep the temperature of the catheter at a safe level below 41°C. For an irradiation time of 10 min under these conditions the patient's fluid load will not exceed 150 ml.

The proximal end of the coaxial cable is connected to a pullback device which moves the emitter along the sheath as the blood vessel is being irradiated. A preprogrammed dose profile is delivered to the adventitia. The length of irradiation can be selected in the range of 0–100 mm. Available irradiation patterns are shown in Figure 20.2. Curve 1 is a simple one, it is created by a continuous movement of the emitter. Curve 2 has two maximums at the ends intended to suppress restenosis beyond stents, the so-called 'candy wrap effect'.

The x-ray system is delivered over a previously positioned standard length guidewire. The marker bands are located at the tip of the sheath at both ends of the guidewire lumen. The emitter is radiopaque and is visible under fluoroscopy. The emitter and cable assembly are advanced to the treatment site, and the treatment is performed over a preprogrammed length. As the irradiation is completed the entire assembly is removed.

Technical specifications

Available sizes	coronary: 1.25 mm, 5-Fr guide catheter and 0.014-inch guidewire compatible (under development) peripheral: 2.2 mm, 7-Fr guide catheter and 0.035-inch guidewire compatible
Emitter's length	5 mm
Radiopacity of emitter	High
Irradiation time for 20-mm lesion	< 10 min
Maximum irradiation length	100 mm
Half-value layer for radiation	1.5–6.0 mm
Operating voltage	20 kV
Operating current	50 μA
Saline flow in the sheath	10–15 ml/min

Why I like the soft x-ray system

- It is an electrical, non-radioactive device. The x-ray radiation is activated on demand by the operator and is always under operator control.
- X-ray devices do not fall under the regulation of the Nuclear Regulatory Commission and can be used in hospitals not licensed for using radioactive materials.
- In contrast to radioactive isotopes the storage, shipping, handling, and disposal of the device are simple.
- The intensity of x-ray radiation does not decrease with time as in the case of radioactive isotopes.
- Penetrating ability of the soft x-ray radiation is optimized; it allows for appropriate irradiation of the vessel wall for prevention of restenosis, but spares the myocardium and pericardium beyond a treatment zone.
- Treatment length is programmable; one device is suitable for lesions of different lengths.
- Irradiation profile along the lesion is programmable; irradiation dose can be increased for areas at the ends of a stent to avoid 'candy wrap' restenosis.
- The catheter is designed as a single operator exchange device; it is flexible and requires only conventional catheter insertion technique.
- Environmentally friendly.

Indications for clinical use

- Native coronary lesions after PTCA with or without stenting
- Native peripheral lesions after PTCA with or without stenting
- Restenotic lesions after PTCA or in-stent restenosis
- Venous bypass grafts

Bibliography

US patent 5,854,822.

21. THE MIRAVANT LIGHT DELIVERY DEVICE FOR PHOTODYNAMIC THERAPY

Miravant Medical Technologies, Santa Barbara, CA, USA

Robert I Grove, Steve Rychnovsky, Pat Stephens, Ian M Leitch, Mark Purter, Ross Heath, Chris Waters and Jeff Walker

Description

A light delivery device for use in the application of photodynamic therapy to prevent restenosis. The device construction is based on existing percutaneous transluminal coronary angioplasty (PTCA) catheter technology with an optical fiber located in the guidewire lumen. The balloon catheter is first placed in position over a guidewire, the guidewire is removed, the fiber is inserted and

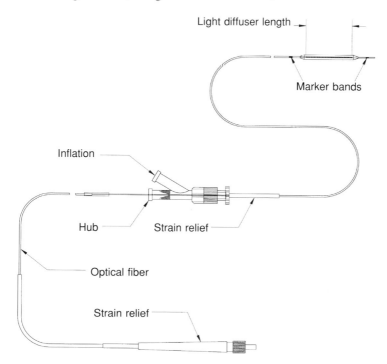

Figure 21.1 *Diagram of Miravant light delivery device.*

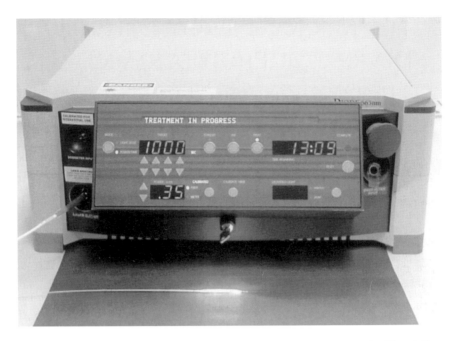

Figure 21.2 Light delivery device connected to a DD2 laser source. The fiber diffuser tip is inserted into the balloon catheter and is emitting 665 nm light from the laser source.

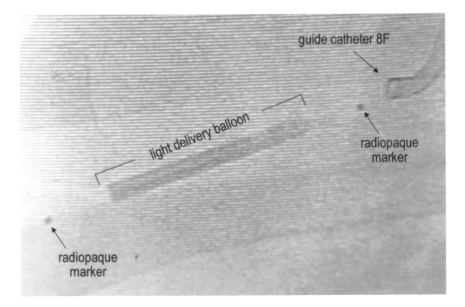

Figure 21.3 Angiogram of light device in swine coronary artery. The diffusing tip of the fiber is centered within the balloon.

168

the balloon is inflated (Figure 21.1). The section of the fiber located within the balloon consists of an optical diffuser element that emits light uniformly (Figure 21.2). The presence of the balloon eliminates optical losses associated with absorption and scattering by blood and also ensures that the diffuser is centered within the artery (Figure 21.3). The proximal end of the fiber is attached to a diode laser (Figure 21.2) capable of emitting a wavelength which activates the photosensitive drug.

Technical specifications	
Light diffuser length	3 cm
Wavelength	665 nm
Balloon diameter	3.0, 3.5, 4.0 mm
Balloon length	4 cm
Balloon material	Nylon
Maximum rated irradiance	300 mW/cm^2
Flexibility	Comparable to PTCA
Trackability	Comparable to PTCA
Radiopaque markers	10 mm proximal and distal to diffuser
Recommended inflation pressure	2 atm
Guidewire compatability	0.014 inch

Indications for clinical use

- Any de novo lesion undergoing PTCA or atherectomy
- Post-PTCA coronary restenosis
- In-stent coronary restenosis
- Peripheral artery restenosis

Tips and tricks

Same as for traditional PTCA balloon catheters.

169

Why I like the PDT system

- Can be placed in any coronary lesion accessible by existing PTCA catheters
- Delivers uniform light dose with a short treatment time
- Utilizes diode laser technology for maximum convenience
- Ensures proper centering of device for uniform treatment
- Eliminates light loss and variability associated with blood absorption
- Minimal penetration of light into surrounding tissue limits side-effects
- The PDT system can be used to treat multiple lesions within a single patient

Review

The ability of photodynamic therapy (PDT) to limit or reduce tumor size by targeting proliferating cells suggested the possibility that the treatment could also be used to inhibit other proliferative diseases. Thus initial studies of PDT in cardiovascular diseases focused on restenosis. In the rat model, systemic administration of a photosensitive drug was followed by a light dose of the correct wavelength to activate the drug. Early studies in rats demonstrated a pronounced PDT-induced effect on intimal hyperplasia that resulted in approximately 90% inhibition.[1-3] The evidence indicated that PDT depleted the vessel wall of smooth muscle cells and suggested that this depletion correlated with inhibition of hyperplasia.[3] In all these early studies the artery was surgically exposed, then irradiated using an external light source.

More recent PDT work in swine utilized intraluminal light delivery techniques. In a study performed in denuded swine iliac arteries, light was administered via an optical fiber positioned at the injury site with the help of a guide catheter.[4] Since this device did not have a balloon element, a continuous saline flush was necessary during light administration to clear blood from the target tissue. Results from this study indicated that PDT exacerbated intimal hyperplasia at 6 weeks in the swine iliac arteries and the possibility of an excessive PDT dose was discussed.[4]

A similar approach was utilized in swine peripheral arteries injured by atherectomy. Following drug administration, an optical fiber with a light diffusing distal end was positioned at the site of the injured artery to deliver the light dose. As in the above case, a saline flush was used to limit absorption by the intervening blood layer. At 21 days, PDT dramatically inhibited hyperplasia.[5] These results are similar to those obtained in rat studies, where

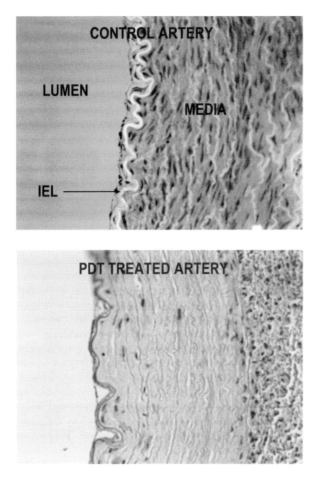

Figure 21.4 PDT-induced acellularity in swine peripheral artery. The artery was harvested 3 days after treatment with the light delivery device in the presence of photosensitive drug. IEL, internal elastic lamina. Note the absence of smooth muscle cells in the medial layer.

PDT was shown to significantly diminish the hyperproliferative response in injured arteries.

Intervention at the coronary level has more rigorous requirements compared with peripheral artery PDT. It is likely that successful PDT in coronary arteries will include devices that are compatible with current angioplasty procedures. Thus it is important that light delivery devices are guidewire compatible and capable of delivering the required light dose in acceptably short periods of time. The Miravant light device was designed to meet these criteria and to be used in the clinic to prevent coronary artery restenosis.

Short-term studies in swine peripheral arteries harvested at 3 days indicated that PDT with the Miravant light device depleted medial smooth muscle cells (Figure 21.4). Early studies in swine coronary arteries demonstrated the ability of the device to deliver appropriate doses of light safely and in acceptably short periods of time in all three coronary arteries (R Waksman, personal communication). Thus, the Miravant light delivery device may have clinical PDT applications in the prevention of post-angioplasty coronary restenosis, as well as in other forms of hyperproliferative vascular disease.

References

1. Ortu P, LaMuraglia GM, Roberts WG, Flotte TJ, Hasan T. Photodynamic therapy of arteries: a novel approach for treatment of experimental intimal hyperplasia. *Circulation* 1992; **85**:1189–1196.

2. LaMuraglia GM, Chandrasekar NR, Flotte TJ, Abbott WM, Michaud N, Hasan T. Photodynamic therapy inhibition of experimental intimal hyperplasia: acute and chronic effects. *J Vasc Surg* 1994; **19**:321–331.

3. Grant WE, Speight PM, MacRobert AJ, Hopper C, Bown SG. Photodynamic therapy of normal rat arteries after photosensitization using disulfonated aluminium phthalocyanine and 5-aminolaevulinic acid. *Br J Cancer* 1994; **70**:72–78.

4. Vincent GM, Fox J, Johnson S, Maragon P. Effects of benzoporphyrin derivative monoacid on balloon injured arteries in a swine model of restenosis. *SPIE* 1996; **2671**:72–77.

5. Gonschior P, Gerheuser F, Fleuchaus M et al. Local photodynamic therapy reduces tissue hyperplasia in an experimental restenosis model. *Photochem Photobiol* 1996; **64**:758–763.

22. THE CL ILLUMINATOR™

Cook Incorporated, Bloomington, IN, USA

Nicholas N Kipshidze, Michael H Keelan Jr and Harry Sahota

Description	Rapid exchange balloon catheter with fiberoptic within the balloon. Fiberoptic has diffuse tip at the distal end. Cold red light is transmitted from a diode laser (650 nm) at energy level 10–150 mW. Figures 22.1 and 22.2 depict the CL Illuminator™ and light source.

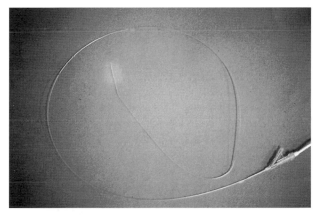

a

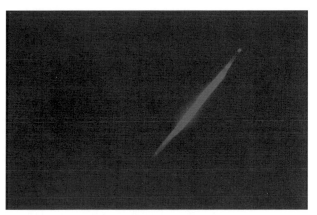

b

Figure 22.1 CL Illuminator™; (a) rapid exchange balloon catheter with fiberoptic within the balloon (b). Note diffuse character of red light.

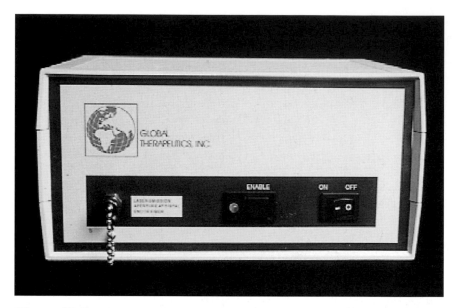

Figure 22.2 *Light source: a diode laser (650 nm) with output power up to 200 mW.*

History	• **1985**	Developing the concept of low power laser light therapy for restenosis (Nicholas Kipshidze)
	• **1992**	Two United States Patents submitted by Drs Nicholas Kipshidze and Harry Sahota
	• **1993–95**	Experience in various animal models
	• **1996**	First clinical use in human coronary arteries, Ivan De Scheerder
	• **1996**	European, Asian and South American clinical trials with CL Illuminator™

Technical specifications

Light source

Light output power	0–100 mW (at the balloon)
Light output wavelength	600–750 nm
Other controls	Internal timer to control dosage; LED display of light activation

Light delivery fiber

	Fiber built into catheter to provide a uniform distribution of light in the radial and axial directions of the balloon

Catheter

Balloon material	PE
Longitudinal flexibility	Excellent
Trackability	Good
Minimal internal diameter of guiding catheter	0.064 inch (6-Fr compatible)
Position of radiopaque markers	Proximal and distal ends of laser light illumination area
Recommended inflation pressure	4–5 atmospheres
Currently available diameters	2.5, 3.0, 3.5 and 4.0 mm
Currently available lengths	20, 30 and 40 mm

Tips and tricks

Same as with conventional PTCA balloon.

Indications for clinical use

• Native coronary lesions
• Recurrent restenosis
• In-stent restenosis
• Venous bypass grafts

Why I like the CL Illuminator™

- Low profile
- Excellent flexibility
- Ability to perform simultaneous PTCA and illumination
- Requires no special training
- Is safe (non-thermal photobiological effect)

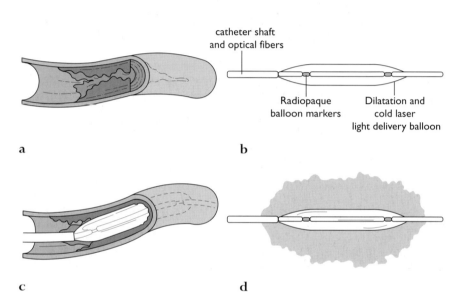

Figure 22.3 *Schematic drawing of the cold laser angioplasty concept. (a) Blocked artery. (b) CL Illuminator™. (c) Angioplasty to open blocked artery. (d) Cold laser light prevents restenosis.*

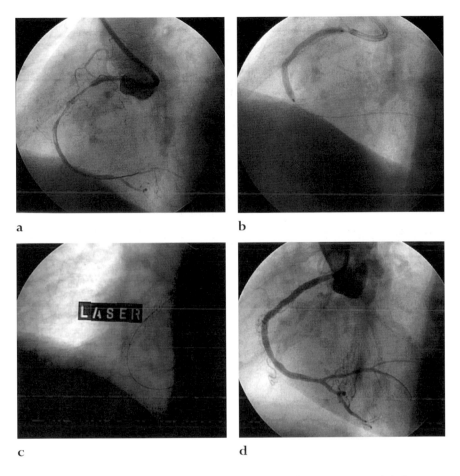

Figure 22.4 *A 76-year-old woman with risk factors of hypertension and diabetes mellitus type II. Reconstruction of RCA with 46-mm stent. Seven months after stent implant, restenosis treated with CL Illuminator™. (By courtesy of Ivan K De Scheerder, MD, PhD, Leuven, Belgium.) (a) Preprocedural angiogram. (b) After 46-mm stent deployment. (c) In-stent restenosis treated with three 1-min IRLI doses. (d) Final outcome 6 months after IRLI. IRLI: intraluminal low-power red laser irradiation.*

Studies	
Past	Non-randomized one-center study
Present	Randomized study—includes two centers in Europe.
	Application towards the end of 2000 to FDA for United States randomized trial in restenotic patients

Review

Coronary artery disease (CAD) remains the most common cause of death in the industrial countries. The introduction of percutaneous transluminal coronary angioplasty (PTCA) in late 1977 began a new era in the management of this disease. Worldwide more than one million patients will undergo PTCA this year. The frequent occurrence of restenosis (40–50%), however, significantly limits the long-term clinical benefits.[1,2]

Experimental studies in animals, postmortem, and intravascular ultrasound data have demonstrated that the biology of restenosis is quite complex. It has been postulated that the process of restenosis has histologic and pathophysiologic similarities to wound healing in other living tissues.[3–5] Endothelial cell (EC) disruption/dysfunction following coronary artery intervention may mediate restenosis, suggesting that rapid regeneration of endothelial cells might impede this process.[6–9]

Numerous reports indicate that non-cytotoxic doses of low-power red laser light (LPRLL) stimulate in vitro cell proliferation and contribute to tissue repair.[10–12] We have observed that LPRLL does enhance endothelial growth as well as attachment in vitro at a dose that has no effect on smooth muscle cell (SMC) proliferation.[13,14] These experiments demonstrated that very low doses of laser irradiation were non-toxic to both EC and SMC. SMC, however, were more resistant to LPRLL, although a higher dose of LPRLL was cytotoxic for both EC and SMC.

Subsequent in vitro studies investigated the effect of LPRLL irradiation on EC and SMC growth.[15] Both rabbit and human EC displayed enhanced growth rate, reaching confluence faster than control non-irradiated cells following laser irradiation with low doses of LPRLL. Higher doses of LPRLL decreased cell growth. In contrast, the experiments on cultured SMC showed that non-toxic doses of LPRLL did not enhance growth in comparison with that of control cultures.

178

The effect of red laser light was then studied in vivo using the balloon injury model in normal rabbit iliac arteries.[14,16] Intravascular laser therapy was applied to one iliac artery following balloon angioplasty, the contralateral artery serving as the control. Animals were sacrificed at 7 days and the extent of endothelialization determined by vital Evans Blue (EB) staining. All vessels undergoing intravascular irradiation remained patent, appeared grossly to be free of thrombus, and failed to take up EB stain. In contrast, three of the control segments showed complete thrombosis and all 10 stained positively with EB. Quantitative analysis identified significant enhancement of re-endothelialization following intravascular LPRLL irradiation. Endothelialization originated from proximal and distal ends of the injured segments in control arteries. In contrast, re-endothelialization was homogeneous throughout the vessel in the laser-treated arteries.

The mechanisms by which laser light enhances endothelial repair were further evaluated by studying the adhesive properties of EC as well as their rate of regeneration. Suspended EC were treated with different doses of red laser light and plated into a 24-well plate. After 3 hours of incubation, Alamar-Blue (AB) assay was performed. It was observed that low doses of light significantly increased the attachment efficiency of EC.[15] Similar results were reported by Karu et al.[17] They demonstrated that low-power red laser stimulates adhesion of He-La cells in vitro and speculated that visible light alters the intensity of ion fluxes through the cell membrane, which may enhance cell sedimentation and adhesion. Functional behavior of tumor cells, however, is not as dependent upon attachment/adhesion, whereas EC require attachment prior to proliferation.

Integrins are major receptors that mediate adhesive interactions in living tissue. They are intimately involved in the regulation of many cellular functions including programmed cell death, hemostasis–thrombosis, leukocyte activation, and the response of cells to mechanical injury.[18] Integrins can trigger several signal transduction pathways and regulate change in gene expression critical for proliferative response and/or affinity of membrane to growth factors. Experimental balloon angioplasty rarely results in complete denudation of endothelium. Based on in vitro (enhancement of cell adhesion) and in vivo (homogeneous endothelialization of entire segment) findings, we feel that intravascular laser therapy may trigger integrin-dependent pathways of preserved endothelium that signal increased DNA synthesis. This results in EC proliferation. We investigated this hypothesis by determining the rate of [³H]thymidine uptake in confluent EC cultures. Low doses of red light increased DNA synthesis by $45.5 \pm 6.8\%$. At higher doses DNA synthesis diminished, consistent with a cytotoxic effect of higher dose therapy.

179

To examine the long-term impact of LPRLL on restenosis using a balloon injury model in the atherosclerotic rabbit, rabbit aortas ($n = 24$/group) were subjected to balloon angioplasty and balloon angioplasty plus intravascular laser illumination.[16] Quantitative angiographic analysis showed that there was no difference in acute gain (0.71 ± 0.06 mm versus 0.61 ± 0.24, $P > 0.05$). Late loss was significantly reduced, however, to 0.14 ± 0.04 mm in the balloon angioplasty plus laser illumination compared with 0.91 ± 0.05 mm in the balloon group ($P < 0.05$). Planimetric and histologic analysis of the harvested arteries revealed that intravascular laser therapy prevented adverse balloon-induced changes, including intimal SMC migration and proliferation.

Although mechanisms by which this might occur have not yet been established, stimulation of endothelial repair with LPRLL may be mediated by integrin-dependent pathways that in turn prevent migration of SMC into media as well as reduction of platelet activation and vascular reactivity.[19,20]

One of the possible mechanisms of the stimulative effect of low-power laser irradiation on endothelial reproduction could be enhanced release of the different growth factors. In vitro experiments in our laboratory indicated that low-power laser irradiation of human SMC in cultured media resulted in a significant increase of secretion of vascular endothelial growth factor (VEGF) measured by sandwich enzyme immunoassay technique. It also was demonstrated that SMC-conditioned media stimulated endothelial cell growth in a dose response manner. This may create a spatial gradient of VEGF towards a denuded area following balloon injury, permitting endothelial cell migration and proliferation. Consistent with this model, LPRLL therapy reduced neointimal hyperplasia in an vivo model.

It may well be that this is one of the mechanisms by which laser energy delivered to ischemic myocardium during the procedure of transmyocardial laser revascularization enhances angiogenesis. Further experimental studies are called for to identify the entire spectrum of mediators and inhibitors that are synthesized and released by vascular cells in response to LPRLL.

We also evaluated the influence of intravascular LPRLL on restenosis in a large animal model.[21] Stents were placed in the right coronary artery of domestic cross-bred pigs. After stent deployment, an additional inflation was performed with the laser-balloon. In group I ($n = 18$), no LPRLL was used; group II ($n = 10$) received an LPRLL dose of 10 mW for 1 min; group III ($n = 10$) received an LPRLL dose of 34 mW for 1 min. Quantitative coronary analysis of the stented vessel was performed before, immediately after stenting, and at 6 weeks. At 6 weeks, the minimal luminal stent diameter was significantly narrower in the control group compared with the LPRLL-treated groups ($P < 0.05$) and late loss correlated inversely proportional to the dose used ($r = 0.9$; $P < 0.03$). These results were confirmed by morphometric analysis. The neointimal area was significantly decreased in the higher dose group. We concluded that intravascular LPRLL contributes to reduction of angiographic restenosis and hyperplastic reaction in this animal model and seems to be dose dependent.

Kipshidze et al[22] reported the long-term results of intraluminal low-power red laser irradiation (IRLI) in 189 patients. All received IRLI using a laser-balloon at a power of 10 mW for three 1-min doses after PTCA and/or stenting procedures. Indications for IRLI were (patients): de novo lesions (37), suboptimal PTCA results (57), bail-out situation (12), bypass graft (2), recurrent restenosis (40), and in-stent restenosis (41). The angiographic characteristics were: mean vessel diameter 3.0 ± 0.7 mm, lesion length 9.3 ± 0.5 mm, type B and C lesions (83.5%), and diffuse disease (32%). No major complications associated with IRLI were observed following interventions and early follow-up.

Angiographic follow-up at 6 months in 71 patients revealed a restenosis (stenosis >50% of luminal diameter) rate in all groups of 16.9%. Moreover, the restenosis rate was only 7.8% in arteries ($n = 38$) with a diameter of ≥ 3.0 mm (late loss index = 0.27 ± 0.1 mm). In arteries ($n = 33$) with a diameter of < 3.0 mm, restenosis occurred in 26% (late loss index = 0.35 ± 0.15 mm). Restenosis in 44 patients with recurrent and in-stent restenosis was 22%.

The authors conclude that IRLI reduces luminal renarrowing in patients following coronary interventions.

References

1. Nobuyoshi M, Kimura T, Nosaka H et al. Restenosis after successful percutaneous transluminal coronary angioplasty: serial angiographic follow up of 229 patients. *J Am Coll Cardiol* 1988; **12**:616–623.

2. Serruys PW, De Jaegere P, Kiemeneij F et al, for the Benestent Study Group. A comparison of balloon-expandable-stent implantation with balloon angioplasty in patients with coronary artery disease. *N Engl J Med* 1994; **331**:489–495.

3. Wolinsky H. Insights into coronary angioplasty-induced restenosis from examination of atherogenesis. *Am J Cardiol* 1987; **60**:65B–67B.

4. Lui M, Roubin G, King S. Restenosis after coronary angioplasty. *Circulation* 1989; **79**:1374–1387.

5. Clowes A, Schwartz S. Significance of quiescent smooth muscle migration in the injured rat carotid artery. *Circ Res* 1985; **56**:139–145.

6. Lüsher TF. The endothelium as a target and mediator of cardiovascular disease. *Eur J Clin Invest* 1993; **23**:670–685.

7. Callow AD, Choi ET, Trachtenberg JD et al. Vascular permeability factory accelerates endothelial regrowth following balloon angioplasty. *Growth Factors* 1994; **10**:223–228.

8. Nabel EG, Plautz G, Boyce FM et al. Recombinant gene expression in vivo within endothelial cells on the arterial wall. *Science* 1989; **249**:1342–1343.

9. Doornekamp F, Borst C, Prost MJ. Endothelial cell recovery and intimal hyperplasia after endothelium removal with or without smooth muscle cell necrosis in the rabbit carotid artery. *J Vasc Res* 1966; **33**:146–155.

10. van Buregel HHFI, Dop Bar PR. Power density and exposure time of He-Ne laser irradiation are more important than total energy dose in photo-biomodulation of human fibroblast in vitro. *Lasers Surg Med* 1992; **12**: 528–537.

11. Karu TI, Pyatibrat LV, Kalendo GS et al. Effects of monochromatic low-intensity light and laser irradiation on adhesions of He-La cells in vitro. *Lasers Surg Med* 1996; **18**:171–177.

12. Lyons RF, Abergel RP, White RA et al. Biostimulation of wound healing in vivo by He-Ne laser. *Ann Plast Surg* 1987; **18**:47–50.

13. Petrosian YS, Kipshidze NN, Putilin SP. Clinical experience with the laser radiation in the treatment atherosclerosis. *Cor Vasa* 1989; **31**:118–121.

14. Kipshidze NN, Keelan MH Jr, Sahota H et al. Biostimulation of wound healing following balloon injury with red laser light in the atherosclerotic rabbit. *J Am Coll Cardiol* 1996; **27**:781.

15. Kipshidze NN, Keelan MH Jr, Horn JB et al. Photobiomodulation of vascular endothelial and smooth muscle cells in vitro with red laser light. *Proceedings – BiOS Europe '96* 1996; 2922.

16. Kipshidze NN, Keelan MH Jr, Nikolaychik V. Impact of red laser light on restenosis. In: Waksman R, King SB, Crocker IR, Mould RF, eds. *Vascular Brachytherapy*. The Netherlands: Nucletron BV, 1996:165–175.

17. Karu TI, Pyatibrat LV, Kalendo GS et al. Effects of monochromatic low-intensity light and laser irradiation on adhesions of He-La cells in vitro. *Lasers Surg Med* 1996; **18**:171–177.

18. Clark EA, Bragge JS. Integrins and signal transduction pathways. The road taken. *Science* 1995; **268**:233–235.

19. Furchgott RF, Ehreich SF, Greenblatt E. The photoactivated relaxation of smooth muscle of rabbit aorta. *J Gen Physiol* 1961; **44**:449–519.

20. Gal D, Chokshi SK, Mosseri M et al. Percutaneous delivery of low-level laser energy versus histamine-induced spasm in an atherosclerotic Yucatan microswine. *Circulation* 1992; **35**:756–768.

21. De Scheerder I, Wang K, Zhou XR et al. Red laser light as adjunct to coronary stent implantation evaluated in a porcine coronary model. *Am J Cardiol* 1997; **80**(7A): 195.

22. Kipshidze N, De Scheerder I, Chevalier B et al. Intraluminal low power red laser therapy: late follow-up *J Am Coll Cardiol* 1998; **31**:236.

23. RADIOCATH™ BRACHYTHERAPY SYSTEM

Mallinckrodt Inc, St Louis, MO, USA

Edward F Smith III

Definition	The RadioCath™ system is an intravascular balloon catheter radiation delivery system filled with a (beta and gamma emitting) radioisotope solution that inflates the balloon catheter to achieve the dosing procedure. The RadioCath system is comprised of four main components: a sodium (Re-186) perrhenate solution in a unit dose glass V-Vial, a radiation shielded manifold transfer device, a radiation treatment balloon (RTB) catheter, and an inflation device.

History	Mallinckrodt designed the RadioCath™ system to minimize deficiencies that limit the overall commercial value of other intravascular brachytherapy systems. The Mallinckrodt RadioCath system was designed to use a PTCA balloon catheter filled with a radioactive solution. This brachytherapy approach was deemed the best, since a balloon catheter system allowed the treatment of both small (i.e. less than 4.0 mm diameter) coronary arteries and larger (i.e. 4–7 mm diameter) peripheral vessels. Additionally, Mallinckrodt was experienced in producing liquid formulation isotopes, especially those suitable for injection for nuclear medicine diagnostic purposes. As a consequence Mallinckrodt was more experienced with injectable radioactivity than medical device companies who saw blood circulating radioactivity as a barrier.
Mallinckrodt has completed 28-day and 6-month studies in pigs subjected to balloon overstretch injury that demonstrate the safety and performance of the RadioCath system.

Technical specifications

- The Re-186 perrhenate component has radiation properties permitting formulation in single-use vials, simplifying product distribution and handling, and minimizing radiation exposure during usage. The liquid in balloon catheter delivers centered dosimetry to vessels of any size and shape, without requiring additional complex device features, enhancing ease of use and improving clinical outcomes.
- In the event of a leak from the balloon catheter, studies in animals and human subjects have demonstrated that perrhenate is cleared rapidly though the kidneys; more than 90% is cleared into the urine in a 24-hour period.
- The shielded manifold transfer device is designed to allow the user to cycle the balloon through multiple inflation and deflation cycles while minimizing radiation exposure.
- The RTB catheter is made of polyethylene material that is more resistant to developing pin-hole leaks. Moreover, the RTB catheter is reinforced with polyethylene terephylate material on the balloon shoulders to provide structural integrity. The rated burst pressure of the RTB is 12 ATM, whereas the inflation pressure is only 5 ATM. This difference between the rated burst pressure and inflation pressure provides a wide margin of safety against potential balloon defects or leaks.
- The RTB catheter is inflated using a Merit Medical Systems Intellasystem™ inflation device. The inflation system has a digital electronic display. The benefit of the system is that it can be programmed to alert the user when the balloon inflation pressure has exceeded the recommended limit, and has the advantage of producing a paper printout depicting the entire inflation pressure and time sequence for insertion into the patient record.

Tips and tricks

The RadioCath system requires the use of the nuclear medicine department. The single use vials are skipped to the nuclear medicine department where they are stored until use. The RTB catheters and shielded manifold are stored in the cath lab where they are available for immediate use. After the angioplasty procedure is completed, the RTB catheter is selected which best matches the diameter of the coronary artery. The RTB catheter is deployed after the angioplasty dilation catheter is removed. Since the RTB is not radiopaque while inflated with the perrhenate solution, it is recommended to inject contrast media down the guide catheter to confirm balloon inflation.

Indications for clinical use

The original intent of the RadioCath program was to evaluate the system for efficacy in preventing restenosis after angioplasty procedures of *de novo* lesions. It is recommended to use the RadioCath system prior to provisional stenting. The RadioCath system is contraindicated in those patients in whom the angioplasty dilation balloon has failed (i.e. leaked or burst) for any reason.

Why I like the RadioCath™ brachytherapy system

The source technology used in the RadioCath™ system (i.e., liquid in balloon catheter) has important market advantages in terms of dosimetry and utility in any vessel. The primary disadvantages of liquid sources all relate to processes for handling radioisotopes. Unlike some of the disadvantages of the alternative radiation sources, Mallinckrodt is confident, as one of the world leaders in nuclear medicine, that these challenges in radioisotope handling can be addressed to the satisfaction of the vast majority of potential customers.

The RadioCath catheter is used in the same manner as a conventional angioplasty balloon catheter. No additional centering devices are required in deploying the RadioCath device. The RadioCath™ balloon catheter is adaptable to different sizes of vessels and lesions, both diameter and length, accessing any portion of a vessel treated by PTCA. The RadioCath™ can be utilized for both coronary artery and peripheral vessel indications. Additionally, intravascular brachytherapy systems with gamma radiation sources require development of special procedures for excessive safety precautions. By comparison, beta radiation from the RadioCath™ posses minimal hazard to medical personnel and standard radiation handling procedures will suffice. The RadioCath system does not require an expensive and elaborate afterloader device (i.e. the dosing table is printed on the package label and the radioactivity emissions are easily shielded without resorting to thick lead shields. Consequently, the attending medical personnel are not required to leave the cath lab to reduce their radiation exposure, and can be at the side of the patient in the event that an emergency situation develops.

Although Re-186 is primarily a beta emitting isotope, it also releases a small amount of gamma radiation, with an energy too low to cause any safety problems, but of sufficient energy to be used to detect the location of Re-186. The values of surveying this gamma emission include the ability to monitor the RadioCath™ treatment and for rapid and precise assessment of spills or leakage.

Relative to other isotopes used in competing intravascular brachytherapy systems, the properties of Re-186 have more favorable aspects for overall product value. The energy of Re-186 is sufficient for efficacy in treating a vessel of any size, peripheral or coronary. In the very rare event of balloon leakage, the rapid metabolic clearance properties of Re-186 perrhenate ensure minimal radiation exposure, compared with isotopes such as P-32 with extensive metabolite reactivity. The 3.7-day half-life of Re-186 is long enough to allow manufacture at a central location and shipment in a simple, single-use vial, making the product available to clinics or hospitals with access to standard radiation handling procedures. On the other hand, because of the much shorter half-life of Re-188 (17 h), brachytherapy systems using this isotope require a commercial generator for on-site production of Rc-188, as well as radiation facilities and staff capable of performing the more sophisticated procedures required for handling generator-produced materials. Currently, very few institutions conducting PTCA procedures have access to the facilities and staff necessary to use a Re-188 brachytherapy system. Furthermore, no commercial Re-188 generator exists, requiring its development and approval by regulatory agencies.

Clinical trials

Mallinckrodt planned two initial pilot trials with the RadioCath device. In December 1998, the MARS I (Mallinckrodt Anti-Restenosis Study) Phase I clinical study was initiated at University Hospital Gasthuisberg (Leuven, Belgium), and Academisch Ziekenhuis, Utrecht, the Netherlands, to evaluate in 60 patients safety and performance of the RadioCath™ system in treating de novo lesions with a single 20 Gy dose to 0.5 mm. Data were collected in these studies for the performance of the entire RadioCath™ system. Included were measurements of the ability to maneuver the balloon to the PTCA-treated lesion, to deliver the appropriate dose and to retrieve the catheter and radioactive solution. A second pilot clinical study, MARS-II, was planned in Canada at sites in Montreal and Toronto. This study aimed to enroll 60 patients randomized to 15 and 20 Gy doses to assess the dose–response requirements.

After 35 patients were enrolled in MARS I, the study was halted temporarily to investigate a leak in the system during a patient treatment. The leak occurred external to the patient and resulted from a laceration on the balloon catheter shaft produced by the incorrect manipulation by the investigator of the balloon shaft with a pair of metal hemostats. Blood and urine samples, and gamma camera imaging after the incident proved negative, confirming the containment of radioactivity outside the patient.

Before the MARS I could be re-started, Mallinckrodt made a strategic decision to stop enrollment in the MARS I study and cancel entirely the MARS II study. The 35 patients enrolled in MARS I will be followed for angiographic follow-up after 6 months. No further clinical activities are planned by Mallinckrodt at this time.

24. EUROPEAN CLINICAL TRIALS

Thoraxcenter, University Hospital Dijkzigt, Rotterdam, The Netherlands

Manel Sabaté, Marco A Costa and Patrick W Serruys

The pioneering work in the field of intravascular radiation therapy was originally carried out in Europe. In 1992. Liermann et al performed the first four cases of brachytherapy after femoral percutaneous angioplasty.[1] Subsequently, animal experiments carried out in the USA[2,3] and Europe[4] demonstrated the reduction of neointimal hyperplasia after endovascular radiotherapy. The insertion of a radioactive delivery catheter in human coronary arteries was performed for the first time by Condado et al in Venezuela.[5] As a result of these pioneering investigations, the first clinical trials were reported in 1997: in the USA, Teirstein et al demonstrated the effectiveness of gamma therapy for the treatment of in-stent restenosis,[6] whilst in Europe, Verin et al reported the feasibility of using beta sources after balloon angioplasty.[7]

In Europe, most of the trials have been carried out using beta-radiation sources, either with catheter-based systems or radioactive stents. Overall, the initial target has been the treatment of de novo coronary stenosis. However, recent design trials have included patients with restenotic lesions. This chapter summarizes the clinical trials carried out in Europe either as a part of larger trials designed in the USA or primarily designed in Europe.

Intracoronary radiation clinical trials using catheter-based systems

The clinical trials with catheter-based systems are summarized in Table 24.1. Initially, these trials were aimed at demonstrating the safety and feasibility of beta emitters in coronary arteries. Currently, results from the dose-finding and placebo-controlled trials are pending.

The GENEVA pilot clinical experience

This was the first feasibility study performed in Europe (Geneva, Switzerland) and also the first in the world to use intracoronary beta-radiation in humans.[7] A pure ^{90}Y beta-emitter source delivered via a centering catheter (Schneider Endovascular Radiation System, Schneider Worldwide, Büllach, Switzerland) was used to deliver 18 Gy at the surface of the balloon in 15 patients with de novo coronary stenoses treated with balloon angioplasty. At follow-up the restenosis rate was 40%. The investigators considered these to be unfavorable results owing to an insufficient dose administered at the adventitia (< 4 Gy).

Table 24.1 Intracoronary radiation clinical trials using catheter-based systems

Study (principal investigator)	Design	Radiation system	Source	Prescribed dose
GENEVA pilot study (V Verin/ Y Popowski)	Prospective, open- label	Schneider intravascular radiation system	^{90}Y wire (29 mm)	18 Gy to the inner arterial surface
Boston Scientific/ Schneider Dose-Finding Study (W Wijns)	Prospective, multi-center, randomized, dose-finding	Boston Scientific/Schneider intravascular radiation system	^{90}Y wire (29 mm)	9, 12, 15, and 18 Gy at 1 mm from the balloon surface
BERT 1.5 – European arm (PW Serruys)	Prospective, uncontrolled	Novoste system	$^{90}Sr/^{90}Y$ seeds (30 mm)	Randomized 12, 14, 16 Gy at 2 mm from the source
Beta Cath (RE Kuntz)	Prospective, randomized, placebo-controlled, triple-masked	Novoste system	$^{90}Sr/^{90}Y$ seeds (30 mm)	Randomized placebo or radiation (14 Gy in vessels ≥ 2.7 ≤ 3.35 mm and 18 Gy in vessels > 3.35 ≤ 4.0 mm) at 2 mm from the source
BRIE (PW Serruys)	Prospective, uncontrolled	Novoste system	$^{90}Sr/^{90}Y$ seeds (30 and 40 mm)	14 Gy ($\geq 2.5 \leq$ 3.25 mm) or 18 Gy ($> 3.25 - \leq 4.0$ mm) at 2 mm from the source
START (JJ Popma)	Prospective, randomized, placebo-controlled triple-masked	Novoste system	$^{90}Sr/^{90}Y$ seeds (30 mm)	Randomized placebo or radiation (16 Gy in vessels $\geq 2.7 \leq$ 3.35 mm and 20 Gy in vessels $> 3.35 \leq$ 4.0 mm) at 2 mm from the source
START 40-20 (JJ Popma)	Prospective, control group of START will be used as control	Novoste system	$^{90}Sr/^{90}Y$ seeds (40 mm)	16 Gy in vessels $\geq$ 2.7 $\leq$ 3.35 mm and 20 Gy in vessels $>$ 3.35 $\leq$ 4.0 mm at 2 mm from the source
RENO (P Urban)	Prospective, surveillance registry	Novoste system	$^{90}Sr/^{90}Y$ seeds (30 and 40 mm)	14–20 Gy after balloon, 16–22 Gy in stented pts, at 2 mm from the source
PREVENT (A Raizner)	Prospective, randomized, blind	Guidant intravascular radiotherapy system/Nucleotron (afterloader)	^{32}P wire (27 mm)	Randomized 0, 28, 35, 42 Gy, at 0.5 mm into the vessel wall

Inclusion	Population/ number of centers	Period	Primary end-point	Status/ results
De novo lesions	15 pts/1 center in Switzerland	June 1995– November 1995	Feasibility and safety at 6 months	Completed — demonstrated safety and feasibility
De novo lesions	181 pts/ 5 centers in Europe	September 1997– September 1999	Angiographic criteria at 6 months	Interim results: dose-dependent reduction in the restenosis rate
De novo lesions	31 pts/ Rotterdam	April 1997–June 1998	Safety, feasibility and angiographic restenosis at 6 months	Completed — demonstrated safety and feasibility
De novo or restenotic lesions without a stent	1450 pts/55 sites in USA and 3 sites in Europe	July 1997–June 2000	TVR and MACE at 8 months	Enrollment phase
De novo or restenotic lesions without a stent in up to two vessels	350 pts (150 pts with single lesions and 100 with 2-vessel disease)/20 sites in Europe	July 1997–June 2000	TVR and MACE at 1 month and 6 months and 1 year. Angiographic criteria, aneurysm formation at 6 months	Enrollment phase
In-stent restenotic lesions	476 pts/49 sites in USA and 2 sites in Europe	September 1998– December 1999	TVR and MACE at 8 months	Follow-up phase
In-stent restenotic lesions	200 pts/25 sites in USA and 1 site in Europe	August 1999– August 2000	TVR and MACE at 8, 12, and 24 months and angiographic restenosis at 8 months	Enrollment phase
De novo or restenotic lesions up to three vessels	1000 pts/50 sites in Europe	April 1999	MACE at 6 months	Enrollment phase
De novo and restenotic lesions	50 pts/site in USA and 35 pts/site in Europe	February 1998–2000	Feasibility, safety and MACE at 1 and 6 months	Enrollment completed: follow-up phase

Continued

Table 24.1 *continued*

Study (principal investigator)	Design	Radiation system	Source	Prescribed dose
INHIBIT (R Waksman)	Prospective, randomized, double-blind, sham-controlled	Guidant intravascular radiotherapy system/Nucletron (afterloader)	^{32}P wire (27 mm)	Randomized 0 or 20 Gy, at 1 mm into the vessel wall
DURABLE (PW Serruys)	Prospective, randomized, controlled, double-blind	Guidant intravascular radiotherapy system/Nucletron (afterloader)	^{32}P wire (27 mm)	16 Gy at 0.5 times reference diameter + 1 mm distance from the source
MARS (De Scheerder)	Prospective, registry	Mallinckrodt system	^{186}Re liquid-filled balloon (25 mm)	20 Gy at 0.5 mm into the vessel wall
GRANITE (PW Serruys)	Prospective, uncontrolled	Cordis gamma IRT™ delivery system	^{192}Ir seeds (23, 39, 55 mm)	14 Gy at 2 mm from the source

Intracoronary beta-radiation following PTCA for reduction of restenosis using the Boston Scientific/Schneider system: Dose-Finding Study

This multi-center, prospective, randomized, non-controlled study aimed to determine the effect of four different doses of beta-radiation, using the ^{90}Y pure beta-emitting source via a centering catheter (Schneider Irradiation Therapy System, Büllach, Switzerland) on coronary stenosis. In five European centers, 181 patients were randomized to receive 9, 12, 15, or 18 Gy at 1 mm tissue depth. The preliminary analysis demonstrated a dose-dependent reduction in angiographic restenosis with an extremely low restenosis rate in the 18 Gy arm: 8.3% in all patients (stented and treated with balloon alone) and 4.2% in patients treated with balloon alone (V Verin, personal communication, Congress of the European Society of Cardiology Barcelona, August 1999). Final results will be available by November 1999.

BERT 1.5 (Beta Energy Restenosis Trial—1.5): the Rotterdam experience

BERT 1.5 stands for the European arm of the BERT trial. This trial was conducted at the Thoraxcenter in Rotterdam in 31 patients from April 1997 to June 1998. This feasibility study was designed to test the ^{90}Sr/^{90}Y source in

Inclusion	Population/ number of centers	Period	Primary end-point	Status/ results
In-stent restenotic lesions	360 pts/USA and Europe	August 1998	TLR, death or Q-MI at 9 months	Enrollment phase
De novo or restenotic lesions (≥ 1 lesion)	900 pts/9 centers in The Netherlands	October 1999	MACE at 1 year	Approval phase
De novo lesions	35 pts/2 centers (Belgium, The Netherlands)	November 1998– March 1999	Feasibility and safety at 6 months	Enrollment completed
In-stent restenotic lesions	120 pts/11 sites in Europe and 1 in Australia	June 1999– February 2003	Angiographic criteria, MACE, safety at 6 and 36 months	Enrollment phase

a hydraulic system (Beta-Cath™ system, Novoste Corporation, Norcross, GA, USA). The dose was randomized to 12, 14 or 16 Gy prescribed at 2-mm depth from the source axis. Twenty-three patients were treated with balloon angioplasty, whereas eight patients received a stent after radiation. Delivery of radiation was successful in all patients but one. At 6 months, the restenosis rate was 28% and target vessel revascularization 23%. Two thrombotic occlusions in patients receiving a stent after radiation were observed at the 2.5- and 10-month follow-up.[14]

Beta-Cath Trial

This prospective, randomized, placebo-controlled trial aims to evaluate the safety and effectiveness of the $^{90}Sr/^{90}Y$ source (Beta-Cath™ system) versus placebo in de novo and restenotic lesions of native coronary arteries. Three centers in Europe are participating in this trial. Complete 8-month follow-up data will be available in 2000.

BRIE Trial (Beta Radiation in Europe)

This non-randomized trial is designed to evaluate the safety and performance of the $^{90}Sr/^{90}Y$ source (BetaCath™ system) in de novo and restenotic lesions of native coronary arteries up to two vessels. This study is being carried out only in Europe (20 sites). Complete 8-month follow-up data will be available in 2000.

START Trial (STents And Radiation Therapy)

This prospective, randomized, placebo-controlled trial aims to evaluate the safety and performance of the $^{90}Sr/^{90}Y$ source (Beta-Cath™ system) in the treatment of in-stent restenosis of native coronary arteries. Two sites in Europe are involved in this study. The enrollment phase will be completed by the end of 1999. One site in Europe will be involved in the START 40-20 Trial, which is designed to assess the feasibility and efficacy of the 40-mm long $^{90}Sr/^{90}Y$ source for the treatment of in-stent restenotic lesions.

RENO Trial (European surveillance Registry with the Novoste Beta-Cath™ system)

This prospective multi-center, multi-national surveillance registry is designed to assess the clinical event rate of $^{90}Sr/^{90}Y$ source (Beta-Cath™ system) combined with approved PTCA techniques (balloon angioplasty, rotablator, laser, and stenting) in patients with coronary artery disease (native or bypass grafts). This study is being carried out only in Europe (50 sites) and multi-vessel treatment up to three vessels is allowed.

PREVENT (Proliferation REduction with Vascular ENergy Trial)

Prospective, randomized, blinded, multi-center study aimed to determine the safety of the Guidant (Santa Clara, CA) beta-radiation system in human coronary arteries following PTCA or stent implantation. The system consists of a ^{32}P 27-mm source wire, a centering spiral balloon and an automatic computerized afterloader (Nucletron BV, Waardgelder, Veenendaal, The Netherlands). The enrollment phase has been completed in Europe and 6-month angiographic and clinical follow-up data are expected by the first quarter of 2000.

INHIBIT (INtimal Hyperplasia Inhibition with Beta In-stent Trial)

A randomized, multi-center, double-blind, sham-controlled study started in the USA and Europe to demonstrate the clinical safety and efficacy of the Guidant beta-radiation system for treatment of in-stent restenosis. The enrollment phase will be completed by the end of 1999 and 9-month angiographic and clinical follow-up will be available by the end of 2000.

DURABLE Trial (DUtch RAndomized Brachytherapy study for Long-term evaluation of Efficacy)

This randomized, placebo-controlled, double-blind study is aimed to assess the effect of brachytherapy by means of the Guidant intravascular brachytherapy system, after optimal balloon angioplasty (stenosis diameter < 35%), elective stenting, and indicated stenting (bail-out and suboptimal result) in patients with multi-vessel stentable lesions (up to two vessels) with respect to MACE-free survival at 1 year. Nine hundred patients will be randomized in nine centers in The Netherlands. The enrollment phase started in October 1999.

MARS (Mallinckrodt Angioplasty Radiation Study)

This is the first European prospective registry to assess the feasibility and safety of the [186]Re liquid-filled balloon (Mallinckrodt System) for the treatment of de novo coronary lesions. Results at the 6-month follow-up will be available by the end of 1999.

The GRANITE Study (Gamma-Radiation to Atheromatous Neointima using Intracoronary Therapy in Europe)

This is the first trial utilizing gamma-radiation for the treatment of coronary in-stent restenosis in Europe. Patients will be followed up for 3 years at 11 sites in Europe including France, Germany, Italy, and The Netherlands, as well as one site in Australia. The radiation system (Gamma IRT™ Delivery System, Cordis, Miami, FL) consists of a ribbon of radioactive ^{192}Ir seeds (up to 55 mm in length) that will be delivered to the target lesion via a delivery catheter with a closed end lumen and using a hand-cranked containment/delivery device. The radioactive ribbon will be left at the angioplasty site for between 15 and 25 min to deliver the prescribed dose.

Intracoronary radiation clinical trials using radioactive stents

The clinical trials utilizing radioactive stents have demonstrated safety and effectiveness in preventing neointimal proliferation in a dose-related manner. However, a new phenomenon has become evident: restenosis at the edges of the high activity radioactive stent, coined the 'candy wrapper' effect.[8] The clinical trials using radioactive stents are summarized in Table 24.2.

IRIS Trial (Isostent for Restenosis Intervention Study)

This feasibility registry involved three centers in Europe in which 40 radioactive stents with an activity of 0.75–1.5 μCi were implanted. This trial demonstrated feasibility and safety with a restenosis rate that ranged between 17% (Rotterdam)[9] and 50% (Milan).[10]

European [32]P Dose–Response Study

This dose-finding study is being conducted in five centers in Europe. Radioactive stents of four ranges of activity have been utilized: 1.5–3.0;

Table 24.2 Intracoronary radiation clinical trials using radioactive stents

Study (principal investigator)	Design	Radiation system	Source	Prescribed dose
IRIS Trial Europe (J Moses)	Prospective, non-randomized	Isostent	32P impregnated Palmaz–Schatz or BX stents (15 mm)	0.75–1.5 μCi
European 32P Dose–Response Study (J Moses)	Prospective, non-randomized	Isostent	32P 15-mm Fischell BX stent	1.5–3.0 μCi, 3.0–6.0 μCi, 6.0–12 μCi, and 12–20 μCi
Cold End Study (J Moses)	Prospective, non-randomized	Isostent	32P 25-mm Fischell BX stent	3–24 μCi in mid 15.9 mm; cold ends 5.7 mm both edges
Hot End Study (J Moses)	Prospective, non-randomized	Isostent	32P 18-mm Fischell BX stent	4.5–9 μCi total activity in mid 14 mm; 2-mm hot ends, 1.3–2.6 μCi/mm

3.0–6.0; 6.0–12; and 12–20 μCi. The Milan group ($n = 82$ patients) reported a suppression of the neointimal hyperplasia in a dose-related manner (between 1.5 and 12 μCi). Edge restenosis ('candy wrapper') was observed in 36% for 1.5–3.0 μCi, 38% for 3.0–6.0 μCi, and 50% for 6.0–12-μCi activity levels.[10] Currently, the Milan group is evaluating the use of stent activities up to 20 μCi.,The Heidelberg group enrolled 11 patients for radioactive stent implantation of activity levels between 1.5 and 3.0 μCi. Target vessel revascularization was 36%, mainly at the articulation of the Palmaz–Schatz stent.[11] In Rotterdam, 40 patients have been evaluated after 6.0–12.0-μCi radioactive stent implantation. To date, 18 patients have returned for angiographic follow-up. No restenosis (> 50% diameter stenosis) was observed within the stent. However, at the edges of the stent the restenosis rate reached 55%, leading to target vessel revascularization in 30% of the patients (AJ Wardeh, personal communication). Data from the Vienna experience will be available at the end of 1999.

Two trials have been designed to address the problem of edge restenosis. The **Cold End Study** is aimed to determine the efficacy and safety of the 32P 25-mm Fischell BX stent, of which both 5-mm ends are inactive ('cold

Inclusion	Population/ number of centers	Period	Primary end-point	Status/ results
De novo or restenotic lesions	40 pts/3 centers (Milan, Rotterdam, Hanover)	September 1997– October 1998	Safety and efficacy on prevention of restenosis at 4–6 months	Completed: demonstrated feasibility and safety
De novo or restenotic lesions	200 pts/5 centers (Milan, Heidelberg, Rotterdam, Aalst, Vienna)	June 1997–ongoing	Safety and efficacy on prevention of restenosis at 4–6 months	Reduction of pure intra-stent restenosis in dose– response manner. Stent edge restenosis $\geq 3\ \mu Ci$
De novo or restenotic lesions	38 pts/3 centers (Rotterdam, Milan, Aalst)	May 1999–ongoing	Safety and efficacy on prevention of restenosis in-stent and at edges at 6 months	Enrollment phase
De novo or restenotic lesions	60 pts/4 centers (Rotterdam, Milan (2 sites), Vienna)	August 1999– ongoing	Safety and efficacy on prevention of restenosis in-stent and at edges at 6 months	Enrollment phase

ends'). Conversely, the **Hot End Study** is aimed to determine the efficacy and safety of the ^{32}P 18-mm Fischell BX stent, of which both 2-mm ends present with higher activity ('hot ends') as compared with the inner 14 mm, which has a total activity ranging from 4.5 to 9 μCi. These two studies are still in the enrollment phase.

Conclusions and future perspective

The use of endovascular beta-radiotherapy in Europe demonstrated that this therapy is safe and feasible. Furthermore, preliminary results of a dose-finding study with the Boston Scientific/Schneider system have been very promising (V Verin, personal communication). This beneficial effect of radiation in preventing restenosis may be explained partially by the positive influence of brachytherapy on the remodeling process.[12,13] However, some detrimental clinical consequences of intracoronary radiation may also be recognized from the European experience. The edge effect, also named 'candy wrapper effect', was

199

reported by Albiero et al after radioactive stent implantation.[10] Further, the occurrence of late coronary thrombosis has been associated with radiotherapy.[14] This phenomenon may be the consequence of delayed endothelialization, persisting dissections[15] or the inability of tubular stents to follow vessel enlargement promoted by radiation leading to late stent malapposition.[16]

Potential solutions for these problems include the use of new designs of radioactive stents or hybrid techniques (catheter-based + radioactive stent)[17] in addition to the use of prolonged antithrombotic therapy. Also, the avoidance of conventional stent implantation may be considered in the setting of catheter-based endovascular radiotherapy.

There are still several unanswered questions which should be resolved before determining the potential of this new technique. First, the use of beta or gamma sources or a combination of both. Secondly, the use of centering or non-centering devices. Further, to determine the best vehicle for radiation: solid (wire or train of seeds), liquid (filled-balloon) or gaseous. Equally, the clinical effect of the dose-rate (radioactive stent—low dose-rate versus catheter-based radiation—high dose-rate). Finally, the target tissue must be defined, as well as the minimal effective dose to be delivered. Hopefully, after the completion of ongoing trials in Europe, as well as in the USA, many of these issues will be answered.

References

1. Liermann DD, Böttcher HD, Kollatch J et al. Prophylactic endovascular radiotherapy to prevent intimal hyperplasia after stent implantation in femoro-popliteal arteries. *Cardiovasc Intervent Radiol* 1994; **17**:12–16.

2. Wiederman JG, Marboe C, Amols H, Schwartz A, Weinberger J. Intracoronary irradiation markedly reduces restenosis after balloon angioplasty in a porcine model. *J Am Coll Cardiol* 1994; **23**:1491–1498.

3. Waksman R, Robinson KA, Crocker IA et al. Intracoronary low-dose β-irradiation inhibits neointima formation after coronary artery balloon injury in the swine restenosis model. *Circulation* 1995; **92**:3025–3031.

4. Verin V, Popowski Y, Urban P et al. Intraarterial beta irradiation prevents neointimal hyperplasia in a hypercholesterolemic rabbit restenosis model. *Circulation* 1995; **92**:2284–2290.

5. Condado JA, Waksman R, Gurdiel O et al. Long-term angiographic and clinical outcome after percutaneous transluminal coronary angioplasty and intracoronary radiation therapy in humans. *Circulation* 1997; **96**:727–732.

6. Teirstein PS, Massullo V, Jani S et al. Catheter-based radiotherapy to inhibit restenosis after coronary stenting. *N Engl J Med* 1997; **336**:1697–1703.

7. Verin V, Urban P, Popowski Y et al. Feasibility of intracoronary beta-irradiation to reduce restenosis after balloon angioplasty. A clinical pilot study. *Circulation* 1997; **95**:1138–1144.

8. Wardeh AJ, Kay IP, Sabaté M et al. Beta particle emitting radioactive stent implantation. A safety and feasibility study. *Circulation* 1999; **100**:1684–1689.

9. Albiero R, Wardeh AJ, DiMario C et al. Acute and 30 day results of 32P β-particle emitting radioactive stent implantation in patients with CAD – The European experience. *Circulation* 1998; **17**:I-778 (abstract).

10. Albiero R, Adamian M, Kobayashi N et al. Acute and intermediate-term results of 32P radioactive β-emitting stent implantation in patients with coronary artery disease. The MILAN dose response study. *Circulation* 1999 (in press).

11. Hehrlein C, Brachmann J, Hardt S et al. P-32 stents for prevention of restenosis: results of the Heidelberg safety trial using the Palmaz–Schatz stent design at moderate activity levels in patients with restenosis after PTCA. *Circulation* 1998; **98**:I-780 (abstract).

12. Sabaté M, Serruys PW, van der Giessen WJ et al. Geometric vascular remodeling after balloon angioplasty and beta-radiation therapy: a three-dimensional intravascular ultrasound study. *Circulation* 1999; **100**:1182–1188.

13. Costa MA, Sabaté M, Serrano P. The effect of P32 beta-radiotherapy on both vessel remodeling and neointimal hyperplasia after coronary balloon angioplasty and stenting. A three-dimensional intravascular ultrasound investigation. *J Invas Cardiol* 1999; **11**: (in press).

14. Costa MA, Sabaté M, van der Giessen WJ et al. Late coronary occlusion after intracoronary brachytherapy. *Circulation* 1999; **100**:789–792.

15. Kay IP, Sabaté M, van Langenhove G. The outcome from balloon-induced coronary artery dissection after intracoronary β-radiation. *Heart* 2000 (in press).

16. Kozuma K, Costa MA, Sabaté M et al. Late stent malapposition occurring after intracoronary beta-irradiation detected by intravascular ultrasound. *J Invas Cardiol* 1999; **11**:651–655.

17. Serruys PW, Kay IP. I like the candy, I hate the wrapper. The ^{32}P radioactive stent. *Circulation* 2000 (in press).

25. US CLINICAL TRIALS

Interventional Technologies, San Diego, CA, USA

Ron Waksman

The ultimate test for any emerging technology to become a standard of care depends on the outcome of the clinical trials. The field of vascular brachytherapy is currently involved in a number of multi-center randomized clinical trials and at the same time data are being collected regarding the long-term outcome of patients who enrolled at early stages of pilot trials. These reports now include 3-year clinical and angiographic information on patients who were treated with intracoronary radiation for the prevention of restenosis and may give a clue to potential side-effects and to the ultimate question as to whether radiation therapy is a panacea to restenosis or only delays restenosis.

Meanwhile new data from larger trials are getting into the pipeline and are being assessed carefully by angiographic and intravascular ultrasound (IVUS) analysis. These studies demonstrate different levels of efficacy and raise new issues regarding dosimetry and complications related to the use of this technology—including the edge effect and late thrombosis phenomenon.

Despite the differences in trial designs, more trials are now focusing on the use of vascular brachytherapy for the prevention of recurrences in patients with in-stent restenosis. The controversies regarding beta- versus gamma-radiation and centering versus non-centering systems are ongoing. Meanwhile, new data related to the use of liquid-filled balloon systems and radioactive stents are being collected.

This chapter summarizes the current status of clinical trials in vascular brachytherapy conducted in the USA.

The peripheral system

The pioneers of the effect of endovascular radiation on restenosis in the peripheral arteries were Liermann and Schopohl from Frankfurt, who initiated a study in 1990 utilizing endovascular radiation in patients with in-stent restenosis at the superficial femoral arteries (SFA). The US clinical trials utilizing vascular radiation for the peripheral arteries are summarized in Table 25.1

Table 25.1 Clinical studies using radiation therapy in the peripheral vascular system

Treated vessel	Principal investigator	Radiation system	Radiation source	Dose (Gy)	Results and status
AV dialysis shunts	Waksman[1]	microSelectron-HDR (Nucletron)	[192]Ir	14	11 patients, 18 lesions, with 40% patency rate at 44 weeks
AV dialysis shunts	Nori[2]	External radiation	Ortho-voltage	8 or 12	15 patients treated in Phase I, 100% occlusion rate at 12 month follow-up
Superficial femoral artery (sponsored by Nucletron-Odelft)	Condado[3] (PARIS trial)	microSelectron-HDR (Nucletron with a centering 7.0 Fr balloon catheter (Guidant)	[192]Ir	14	Phase I registry of 40 patients completed, demonstrated safety and lower restenosis rate of 12% at 6 months Phase II multicenter, double-blind, randomized study in 300 patients has been initiated

PARIS (Peripheral Arteries Radiation Investigational Study) is a US multi-center, randomized, double-blind control study in 300 patients following percutaneous transcatheter angioplasty (PTA) to SFA stenosis using a gamma-radiation ^{192}Ir source. The treatment dose is 14 Gy delivered via a centered segmented end lumen balloon catheter utilizing the microSelectron-HDR (Nucletron) afterloader. The objectives of this study are to determine angiographic evidence of patency and reduction of > 30% of the restenosis rate of the treated lesion at 6 months. A secondary end-point is to determine the clinical patency at 6 and 12 months by treadmill exercise and by the ankle-brachial index (ABI). The feasibility study of 40 patients in this trial was completed with clinical success of the brachytherapy procedure in 35 of the patients, with no reports of adverse events related to the radiation therapy and encouraging angiographic restenosis of < 12% in the target vessel at 6 months.[1] The randomized phase was initiated in 1998 in 15 centers and enrollment should be completed at the end of 2000.

204

Arteriovenous dialysis graft

Studies on the treatment of patients with arteriovenous (AV) dialysis graft stenosis utilizing external radiation therapy have been launched by Nori et al.[2] The first 10 patients were treated successfully with a fractionated total dose of 8 or 12 Gy. There were no reports on procedure-related complications. Within a year of radiation treatment, all patients in this cohort required intervention because of graft failure.

A pilot trial to attempt to reduce the recurrence rate in patients with AV dialysis grafts by endovascular radiation, using the microSelectron-HDR afterloader and a non-centering catheter, demonstrated feasibility in 12 treated grafts, but only 40% of grafts remained open at 12 months.

Other targets for radiation therapy are renal arteries and following transjugular intrahepatic porto-systemic shunting (TIPS) procedures.

The coronary system

Various pilot studies with intracoronary brachytherapy have examined the feasibility and safety of this technology with new systems, using a variety of emitters. A summary of the clinical trials conducted so far with gamma and beta emitters is given below. Clinical trials utilizing gamma- and beta-radiation are listed in Tables 25.2 and 25.3, respectively.

Gamma-radiation trials

The first clinical trial using intracoronary radiation in human coronary arteries was conducted by Condado et al,[3] and 3-year angiographic and clinical outcomes were reported recently. In this study, 21 patients (22 arteries) with unstable angina underwent PTCA followed by intracoronary radiation with ^{192}Ir (19–55 Gy). Repeat angiography at 30–60 days demonstrated total occlusions in two arteries, a new pseudoaneurysm in one artery and significant dilatation at the treatment site of two additional arteries. The remaining arteries were patent. At the 6-month follow-up, all remaining arteries (20) were patent with a loss index of 0.19. More recently, the 2- and 3-year angiographic results have shown a binary restenosis of 28% with a loss index of 0.26, with no adverse events.[4] In addition, there was no evidence of any clinical adverse events related to radiation in these patients at 4 years.

SCRIPPS (Scripps Coronary Radiation to Inhibit Proliferation Post Stenting) was the first randomized trial on the safety and efficacy of intracoronary gamma-radiation given as adjunct therapy to stents to reduce coronary restenosis. In this study, 55 patients were randomized to receive placebo or ^{192}Ir (8–30 Gy, dosimetry guided by IVUS) utilizing a ribbon (19–35 mm)

Table 25.2 US clinical trials using catheter-based systems with gamma-radiation [192]Ir.

Principal investigator (Sponsor)	Study name and design	Radiation system	Dose (Gy)	Results and status
Condado[4] (Angiorad)	Open-label, radiation following balloon angioplasty in 21 patients (22 native coronary arteries)	Hand delivered 0.014" or 0.018" 30-mm iridium wire into a non-centered 4.0 Fr closed end lumen catheter (Angiorad)	20 and 25: actual doses 19–55	Completed. Clinical and angiographic follow-up at 8 and 36 months demonstrated safety and low late loss indices
Teirstein[6] (Best Medical)	SCRIPPS: single-center double-blind randomized in 55 patients with restenosis and stenting	Hand delivered 0.030" nylon ribbon with seeds (Best Medical) into a closed end lumen non-centered 4.5 Fr catheter (Navius)	≥8–<30 to media by IVUS	Completed. Reduction of restenosis in the irradiated group by clinical, IVUS and angiograms at 6 months
Waksman[7] (CRF, WHC)	WRIST (native coronaries): single-center double-blind randomized in 130 patients with in-stent restenosis	Hand delivered 0.030" nylon ribbon with seeds (Best Medical) into a non-centered closed end lumen 5.0 Fr catheter (Medtronic)	15 at 2.0 mm for vessels 3–4 mm	Significant reduction in restenosis rate (67%) and the need for revascularization (63%)
Waksman[7] (CRF, WHC)	SVG WRIST: multi-center double-blind randomized in 120 patients with in-stent restenosis	Hand delivered 0.030" nylon ribbon with seeds (Best Medical) into a non-centered closed end lumen 5.0 Fr catheter (Medtronic)	15 at 2.4 mm for vessels >4.0 mm	Initial results in 30 patients from WRIST showed reduction in restenosis in the irradiated vein grafts
Waksman* (CRF, WHC)	Long WRIST (36–80 mm): two-center double-blind randomized in 120 patients with in-stent restenosis	Hand delivered 0.030" nylon ribbon with seeds (Best Medical) into a non-centered closed end lumen 5.0 Fr catheter (Medtronic)	15 at 2.0 mm for vessels 3–4 mm	Enrollment completed in July 1999, data will be available in spring of 2000
Waksman* (CRF, WHC)	Long WRIST High Dose (36–80 mm): two-center registry of 60 patients with in-stent restenosis	Hand delivered 0.030" nylon ribbon with seeds (Best Medical) into a non-centered closed end lumen 5.0 Fr catheter (Medtronic)	15 at 2.4 mm for vessels 3–4 mm	Enrollment started January 1998, study will be completed in 2000

Table 25.2 *continued*

Principal investigator (Sponsor)	Study name and design	Radiation system	Dose (Gy)	Results and status
Waksman* (CRF, WHC)	WRIST Plus (Plavix for 6 months): single-center registry of 120 patients with in-stent restenosis in native and vein grafts	Hand delivered 0.030" nylon ribbon with seeds (Best Medical) into a non-centered closed end lumen 4.0 Fr catheter (Cordis)	14 at 2.0 mm for vessels 2.5–4.0 mm	Enrollment started July 1999, angiographic follow-up at 6 months will determine the late thrombosis rate
Leon[8] (Cordis)	GAMMA 1: multi-center double-blind randomized in 250 patients with in-stent restenosis	Hand delivered 0.030" nylon ribbon with seeds (Best Medical) into a non-centered closed end lumen 4.0 Fr catheter (Cordis)	≥8–<30 to media by IVUS	Study completed, demonstrated reduction of restenosis and TLR in the irradiated group vs control
Leon* (Cordis)	GAMMA 2: multi-center open-label registry of 125 patients with in-stent restenosis	Hand delivered 0.030" nylon ribbon with seeds (Best Medical) into a non-centered closed end lumen 4.0 Fr catheter (Cordis)	14 Gy at 2 mm for vessels 2.5–4.0 mm	Enrollment was completed in summer 1999, data will be available in summer 2000
Faxon[?] (Vascular Therapies)	ARREST: double-blind randomized in 700 patients post-PTCA and provisional stenting	Mechanical delivery of 0.014" fixed wire 30 mm (Angiorad) into a monorail closed end lumen balloon centering 3.2 Fr catheter	<8–<35 to media by IVUS	Feasibility phase completed, restenosis rate of 40%, multi-center phase is pending
Waksman[10] (Vascular Therapies)	ARTISTIC: multi-center double-blind randomized in 290 patients with in-stent restenosis	Mechanical delivery of 0.014" fixed wire 30 mm (Angiorad) into a monorail closed end lumen balloon centering 3.2 Fr catheter	12, 15 or 18 to 2.0 mm distance	Feasibility phase completed, with low restenosis rate (13%) multi-center initiated in the summer of 1998
Waksman* (CRF)	SMARTS: double-blind, randomized in 180 patients with small vessels (2.00–2.75 mm) with provisional stenting	Mechanical delivery of 0.014" fixed wire 30 mm (Angiorad) into a monorail closed end lumen balloon centering 3.2 Fr catheter	12 to 2.00 mm distance from the source	Study initiated in the fall of 1998 and ongoing, depending on current supplies of the system

*Data not available at time of writing.

Table 25.3 US clinical trials using catheter-based systems with beta-emitters in coronaries

Principal investigator (Sponsor)	Study name and design	Radiation system	Isotope and dose (Gy)	Results and status
King[11] (Novoste)	BERT: open-label in 23 patients post-PTCA in de novo lesions	Hydraulic hand delivery of a train of 12 radioactive seeds (30 mm) in a non-centered 5.0 Fr catheter	^{90}Sr/Y, 12, 14, 16 Gy to 2 mm from source	Completed; demonstrated feasibility, safety, restenosis rate of 15% with late loss of 0.05 mm and loss index of 4%
Kuntz* (Novoste)	Beta-Cath: multi-center, randomized, blinded study in 1100 patients after PTCA and provisional stenting	Novoste Beta-Cath system	^{90}Sr/Y, 14, 18 Gy to 2 mm from source	Study initiated in July 1997, currently conducted in 25 centers in the USA
Raizner[12] (Guidant)	PREVENT: multi-national open-label feasibility study in 80 patients after PTCA or stenting (Phase I)	Automatic afterloader (Nucletron) of 0.018" 27-mm fixed wire via a helical centering balloon, 2.5–4.0 mm, 30 mm length	^{32}-P 16, 20 or 24 Gy to 1.0 mm from the source	Enrollment completed in May 1998, demonstrated safety at 30 days, lower late loss and target lesion revascularization (TLR) in the irradiated group; multicenter randomized blinded study to follow
Weinberger[13] (Columbia University)	CURE: registry open-label in 30 patients post-PTCA and 30 before stenting	Liquid ^{188}Re from a generator (Oak Ridge) fills a perfusion coronary balloon, Lifestream™	^{188}Re, 13 Gy to the vessel wall	Initiated in October 1997, enrollment of 30 patients was completed, reported TLR of 17%
Waksman* (CRF)	Beta WRIST: registry for 50 patients with in-stent restenosis	Schneider System ^{90}Y source centering balloon and an afterloader	20.6 Gy to 1.0 mm distance from source	Enrollment was completed in June of 1998, acute safety was demonstrated at 30 days
Waksman* (CRF)	INHIBIT: multi-center for patients with in-stent restenosis, for 320 patients	Automatic afterloader (Nucletron) 0.018" 27-mm fixed wire via a helical centering balloon	^{32}P, 20 Gy to 1.0 mm from source	Study was initiated in June 1998

Table 25.3 *continued*

Principal investigator (Sponsor)	Study name and design	Radiation system	Isotope and dose (Gy)	Results and status
Hueser* (Novoste)	START: multi-center double-blind controlled study for 400 patients with in-stent restenosis	Novoste Beta-Cath system, lesions up to 20 mm in length treated with 30-mm source train	[90]Sr/Y, 16–20 Gy at 2 mm from the source	Study initiated in September 1998; enrollment completed and results will be available in spring of 2000
Hueser* (Novoste)	START 40/20: multi-center registry for 200 patients with in-stent restenosis	Novoste Beta-Cath system, lesions up to 20 mm in length treated with 40-mm source train	[90]Sr/Y, 16–20 Gy at 2 mm from source	Enrollment was completed in October 1999; results will be available in the summer of 2000
Waksman (CRF)	R²: rotablation and radiation randomized double-blind study in de novo or restenotic lesions	Schneider/Boston Scientific system, ^{90}Y source, centering balloon and an afterloader; following rotablator	20.6 Gy to 1.0 mm distance from source	Study pending on FDA approval

*Data not available.

delivered in a non-centered closed end lumen catheter at the treatment site (dwell time 20–45 min). This study demonstrated 6-month angiographic restenosis in 17% versus 54% in the placebo group. No clinical complications resulting from the radiation treatment were evident, and the clinical benefits were maintained at 3 years with a significant reduction in the need for target lesion revascularization at 3 years, $P = 0.004$.[5,6]

WRIST (Washington Radiation for In-stent Restenosis Trial)[7] is a series of studies designed to evaluate the effectiveness of radiation therapy for in-stent restenosis. In the first study, 130 patients (100 patients with native coronary arteries and 30 patients with vein grafts) with in-stent restenosis lesions (up to 47 mm in length) were randomized blindly to treatment with either placebo or radiation. The source was ^{192}Ir and the prescribed dose was 15 Gy at 2 mm from the source into the vessel wall. At 6 months the clinical and angiographic follow-up showed a dramatic reduction of the restenosis rate: 19% in the irradiated group versus 58% in the control group. There was a

79% reduction in the need for revascularization and a 63% reduction in major cardiac events (death, Q-wave myocardial infarction, and any revascularization) in the irradiated group compared with controls. Intravascular ultrasound sub-analysis demonstrated regression of tissue in 53% of the irradiated arteries at follow-up. This study is considered a landmark in the establishing of gamma-radiation for the treatment of in-stent restenosis.

Long WRIST is a two-center randomized double-blind control study to examine the effectiveness of the same system and dose used in WRIST in long lesions (36–80 mm) in 120 patients.

Long WRIST High Dose is a registry of 60 patients with the same inclusion/exclusion criteria as Long WRIST for vessels up to 4 mm in diameter; the prescribed dose is 15 Gy at 2.4 mm from the source.

SVG WRIST is a multi-center randomized double-blind control study using the same system and protocol as above for 120 patients with in-stent restenosis in vein grafts.

WRIST Plus is a single-center registry of 120 patients with similar inclusion/exclusion criteria to all the WRIST studies. The main objectives of this study are to determine whether long-term antiplatelet therapy (Clopidogrel 75 mg/q.d. for 6 months) will reduce the late thrombosis phenomenon.

GAMMA 1 is a multi-center, randomized double-blind trial in which 250 patients are being enrolled for treatment for in-stent restenosis with a hand-delivered ^{192}Ir ribbon source while the dosimetry is guided by intravascular ultrasound (doses between 8 and 30 Gy). Recently the 6-month angiographic results were presented, showing significant reduction in the in-stent angiographic restenosis rate in the radiation arm: 21.6% versus control 52%. Sub-analysis for lesion length demonstrated a 70% reduction in angiographic restenosis for lesions < 30 mm in length versus a reduction of only 48% for lesions between 30 and 45 mm in length.[8] In addition, the edge effect was noted in patients who had not had enough coverage of the lesion by the radioactive seeds.

ARTISTIC (Angiorad Radiation Technology for In-Stent restenosis Trial In native Coronaries) is a study in which a 0.014-inch fixed 30-mm ^{192}Ir wire is being used in a blinded, randomized manner in 300 patients with in-stent restenosis in native coronary arteries. The pilot phase of the study in 26 patients was recently completed and 6-month angiographic follow-up was reported to show low binary restenosis rates of 10%, lower late loss index of 0.12 and lower major cardiac adverse events of 15%.[10]

ARREST (Angiorad Radiation for REstenosis Trial), a multi-center pilot study in 25 patients, was completed recently. Patients enrolled with de novo or restenotic lesions that were treated with balloon angioplasty alone and then with open-label radiation therapy using the Angiorad radiation system with a fixed ^{192}Ir wire source and dosimetry based on IVUS findings. The pilot study demonstrated feasibility and safety. However, the angiographic restenosis rate in this feasibility cohort was 45% and was explained by underdosing the target area (< 8 Gy to the adventitia).[9]

SMARTS (SMall Artery Radiation Therapy Study) is a randomized trial in 180 patients with small vessel disease (2.0–2.75 mm) treated with gamma-radiation (^{192}Ir).

Beta-radiation trials

Clinical trials using beta emitters were initially designed to examine the effectiveness of beta-radiation therapy for prevention of restenosis for de novo lesions in native coronary arteries. Later studies have been initiated to test the effectiveness of beta-radiation for in-stent restenosis.

BERT (Beta Energy Restenosis Trial) is a feasibility study approved by the FDA limited to 23 patients in two centers (Emory and Brown Universities). The study was designed to test the ^{90}Sr/^{90}Y source delivered by a hydraulic system (Novoste, Norcross, GA, USA). The prescribed doses in this study were 12, 14, or 16 Gy and the treatment time did not exceed 3.5 min. The radiation was successfully delivered to 21 of 23 patients following conventional PTCA with no complications or adverse events at 30 days. At follow-up, two patients at 6 months and one patient at 9 months underwent repeat revascularization to the target lesion.[11] The Canadian arm of this study included 30 patients from the Montreal Heart Institute and the European arm (BERT 1.5) was conducted at the Thoraxcenter in Rotterdam in an additional 30 patients, utilizing the same system under the same protocol and had a reported restenosis rate of 25%. At 6-month follow-up the level of angiographic restenosis for the entire cohort of 84 patients was 17%, with lower rates of late loss at 9%. However, six more patients required revascularization owing to edge effect.

The Beta-Cath trial was initiated in July 1997 as a prospective, randomized, placebo-controlled trial to evaluate the safety and effectiveness of the ^{90}Sr/[90]Y Beta-Cath system versus placebo in de novo or restenotic lesions of native coronary arteries. A total of 1100 patients undergoing elective PTCA or provisional stent placement has been enrolled in > 35 centers and the angiographic follow-up at 8 months will be available by the spring of 2000. A further 300 patients were added to the stent arm of the study because of the higher rates of late thrombosis observed in one of the treated groups, which required a change in the antiplatelet protocol. The results of this study will determine the use of this technology for prevention of restenosis for de novo lesions.

PREVENT (Proliferation Reduction with Vascular Energy Trial) is a prospective, randomized, blinded, multi-national, multi-center study; its objective is to demonstrate the safety of the Guidant (Santa Clara, CA, USA) beta-radiation system in human coronaries immediately following PTCA or a stent placement. The system consists of ^{32}P isotope, 27 mm in length, delivered into a centering helical balloon delivery catheter via an automatic afterloader apparatus. The doses in this open-label phase are 16, 20 and 24 Gy, prescribed to 1 mm from the source. The feasibility phase of the study was completed in May 1998 and the preliminary results suggested low rates of late loss in the irradiated group (4.8% compared with control 51.3%) with significant reduction in the need for target lesion revascularization (4% versus 18%). However, owing to an increase of edge effect the target lesion revascularization rates were similar in the treated vessels (24% versus control 29%).[12] Sub-analysis of patients with in-stent restenosis treated with ^{32}P demonstrated lower rates of recurrences—20% compared with a matched control group from the WRIST study (66%).

CURE (Columbia University Radiation Energy) is the first liquid-filled balloon system to be used in a feasibility clinical trial and includes 30 patients who have had balloon angioplasty or 30 patients undergoing intracoronary stenting. The study has been initiated in Columbia University (New York City, NY) under an institutional IDE. The isotope in the liquid form is ^{188}Re retrieved from a 188-tungsten generator injected via syringe into a perfusion balloon (Lifestream™, Guidant) to allow a dwell time of up to 10 min. No data on the feasibility and the safety of this system have been reported yet. Target lesion revascularization was reported in 5 of the 30 patients treated in this cohort (17%).[13]

Beta-radiation trials for in-stent restenosis lesions

Studies to examine the effectiveness of beta-radiation systems in preventing recurrence of in-stent restenosis have been launched, including Beta WRIST (^{90}Y), INHIBIT (^{32}P) and START (^{90}Sr/Y). These are similar in design and aim to address the efficacy of beta emitters for the treatment of restenosis in order to expedite approval for marketing in the USA.

Beta WRIST is the first study to report on the efficacy of beta-radiation for prevention of in-stent restenosis. This is a registry of 50 patients undergoing treatment for in-stent restenosis in native coronary arteries and treated with a beta-radiation system using the yttrium-90 source, a centering catheter and an afterloader system. The clinical outcome of these patients was compared with the control group of the original cohort of WRIST who were randomized to placebo versus ^{192}Ir. In Beta WRIST, the reported angiographic restenosis rate at 6 months was 22%, about 10% of the patients had late thrombosis. Overall the use of beta-radiation for the treatment of in-stent restenosis demonstrated a reduction of > 50% in the need for target lesion or vessel revascularization compared with the historical control of WRIST.[14] Comparison of the outcome of the beta-radiation group with the gamma-radiation group did not detect major differences between these two groups. This study suggested that treatment for in-stent restenosis with beta emitters may have a similar outcome to that shown for gamma emitters.

START (Stents and Radiation Therapy)

This is an FDA pivotal multi-center, randomized trial in over 55 centers in the USA and Europe which will determine the efficacy and safety of the Beta-Cath system for the treatment of in-stent restenosis. The doses in this trial are 16 and 20 Gy at 2 mm from the center of the source, depending on vessel diameter. The enrollment of 385 patients has been completed and results will be available in the spring of 2000.

START40/20. This is a registry of 200 patients in the USA to determine the efficacy of longer source trains for the treatment of lesions up to 20 mm. Inclusion/exclusion criteria for this study are similar to those for the START study.

INHIBIT. This is a multi-center randomized study taking place in the USA and Europe for patients with in-stent restenosis to test the efficacy of the Galileo system using a ^{32}P source with a dose of 20 Gy at 1 mm from the surface of the balloon. The antiplatelet therapy for this study is prescribed for 3–6 months and all patients will undergo angiographic follow-up at 8 months. The study was initiated in July of 1998 and enrollment will be completed by December 1999.

So far the lessons learned from the beta feasibilitiy studies show that the radiation effect is confined to the length of the source and longer beta sources are required to cover the entire segment undergoing intervention to eliminate the edge effect phenomenon.

Radioactive beta-emitting stents

Clinical trials with the radioactive stent have demonstrated safety, but were disappointing in efficacy. The isotope examined on this radioactive stent was ^{32}P and the platform was either the Palmaz–Schatz PS 153, or the BX stent.

IRIS (Isostent for Restenosis Intervention Study) was the first feasibility study using the radioactive ^{32}P Palmaz–Schatz stent (Isostent, San Carlos, CA, USA). In this study, 30 patients with stenosis in de novo or restenotic lesions of native coronary arteries underwent radioactive stent implantation (activity between 0.5 and 1.0 μCi). There were no adverse effects at 30 days in any of the treated patients; however, at 6-month angiographic follow-up there was a binary restenosis rate of 31% and clinical driven target lesion revascularization of 21%. Late loss data by segment were 0.94 mm for de novo and 0.70 mm for restenosis lesions. IVUS detected a significant amount of diffuse disease, with a mean CSA stenosis of 41% in the reference vessel at the time of the stent implantation.[15]

The IRIS trial was expanded for an additional 25 patients who underwent intracoronary stent implantation with higher activity (0.75–1.5 µCi) stent (mean activity 1.14 µCi). This cohort demonstrated safety of the radioactive stent without evidence of thrombus or subacute closure, but the overall restenosis rate was higher than that reported for a non-radioactive stent.[16]

References

1. Waksman R, Laird JR, Benenati J et al. Intravascular radiation for prevention of restenosis after angioplasty of narrowed femoral-popliteal arteries: Preliminary six month results of a feasibility study. *Circulation* 1998; **98**:66:331.

2. Nori K. External radiation for AV-dialysis fistulas: results from pilot studies (abstract). *Advances in Cardiovascular Radiation Therapy III*. Washington, DC, Feb 17–19, 1999.

3. Condado JA, Waksman R, Gurdiel O et al. Long-term angiographic and clinical outcome after percutaneous transluminal coronary angioplasty and intracoronary radiation therapy in humans. *Circulation* 1997; **96**:727–732.

4. Condado JA, Saucedo JF, Caldera C et al. Two year angiographic evaluation after intracoronary 192 Iridium in humans. *Circulation* 1997; **96**:I-220.

5. Teirstein PS, Massullo V, Jani S et al. Catheter-based radiotherapy to inhibit restenosis after coronary stenting. *N Engl J Med* 1997; **336**:1697–1703.

6. Teirstein PS, Massullo V, Jani S et al. Two-year follow-up after catheter-based radiotherapy to inhibit coronary restenosis. *Circulation* 1999; **99**:243–247.

7. Waksman R, White RL, Chan RC et al. Intracoronary radiation therapy for patients with in-stent restenosis: 6-month follow-up of a randomized clinical study. *Circulation* 1998; **98**:17,I-651:3421.

8. Leon MB, Teirstein PS, Lansky AJ et al. Intracoronary gamma radiation to reduce in-stent restenosis: the multicenter Gamma I randomized clinical trial. *J Am Coll Cardiol* 1999; **33**:56A (abstract).

9. Faxon DP, Buchbinder M, Cleman MW et al. Intracoronary radiation to prevent restenosis in native coronary lesions: the results of the pilot phase of the ARREST trial. *J Am Coll Cardiol* 1999; **33**:19A (abstract).

10. Waksman R, Porrazzo MS, Chan RC et al. Results from the ARTISTIC feasibility study of 192-iridium gamma radiation to prevent recurrence of in-stent restenosis. *Circulation* 1998; **98**:17,I-442:2327.

11. King SB, Williams DO, Chougule P et al. Endovascular beta-radiation to reduce restenosis after coronary balloon angioplasty. Results of the beta energy restenosis trial (BERT). *Circulation* 1998; **97**:2025–2030.

214

12. Raizner AE, Oesterle S, Waksman R et al. The PREVENT trial, a feasibility study of intracoronary brachytherapy in the prevention of restenosis: An interim report. *Circulation* 1998; **98**:I-651 (abstract).

13. Weinberger J. Clinical experience with the liquid-filled balloon: The CURE Study (abstract). *Advances in Cardiovascular Radiation Therapy III*, Washington, DC, Feb 17–19, 1999.

14. Waksman R, White RL, Chan RC et al. Intracoronary beta radiation therapy for in-stent restenosis: preliminary report from a single center clinical study. *J Am Coll Cardiol* 1999; **33**:19A (abstract).

15. Baim DS, Fischell T, Weissman NJ, Laird JR, Marble SJ, Ho KK. Short term (1 month) results of the IRIS feasibility study of a beta particle emitting radioisotope stent. *Circulation* 1997; **96**:I-218.

16. Moses J. US IRIS low-activity ^{32}P stent (abstract). *Advances in Cardiovascular Radiation Therapy III*, Washington, DC, Feb 17–19, 1999.

26. ENDOVASCULAR BRACHYTHERAPY SAFETY TIPS

Lenox Hill Hospital Heart and Vascular Institute of New York, NY, USA

Stephen Balter

Introduction

Staff risks from conventional fluoroscopy and endovascular brachytherapy (EVBT) can be minimized by appropriate attention to the usual principles of radiation safety. This chapter reviews specific EVBT radiation safety issues under normal and emergency conditions. One expects a minimum of technical emergencies. Contingency plans must be made, discussed, and rehearsed for a variety of likely and unlikely occurrences. Some representative events are described in this paper without estimating their frequency.

The goal of any safety program is to keep risks within both regulatory and personally acceptable limits. Increasing patient safety and efficacy might increase staff risk. Certain combinations of radiation sources and treatment devices minimize or eliminate staff dose. However, the safest combination, from a staff member's point of view, may or may not deliver the most effective treatment to the patient. Balancing patient benefit and staff risk is a common ethical situation.

Natural background radiation levels are 3 millisievert per year (mSvy^{-1}: 300 millirems per year) in New York City and 4 mSvy^{-1} in Denver. Regulatory authorities currently specify a maximum permissible dose (MPD) of 1 mSvy^{-1} for members of the public and 50 mSvy^{-1} for radiation workers. The NCRP recommends that any worker's effective dose average is < 10 mSvy^{-1}. The ICRP's corresponding value is 20 mSvy^{-1}. The 'as low as reasonably achievable' (ALARA) principle motivates dose reduction to levels significantly below the MPD.

Physics review

The dose-rate delivered by a radioactive source depends on both the activity of the source and the radionuclide that it contains. The same activity of two different nuclides can deliver dose-rates that differ by a factor of > 10.

All removable EVBT sources deliver energy at high dose-rate (HDR). Safety concerns and operating procedures differ for HDR sources in comparison with low dose-rate (LDR) sources such as radioactive stents.

The total dose delivered by a source depends on its initial activity, its radioactive decay properties, and the time that it is in position. Over time, small permanently implanted LDR sources deliver larger doses to the target than large HDR sources. The radiobiological reasons for this requirement are beyond the scope of this chapter.

Bremsstrahlung (braking radiation) is formed when high-energy electrons (e.g. beta particles) interact with matter. In fact, this is the primary mechanism of x-ray production in an x-ray tube. The physical behavior of a bremsstrahlung photon is identical to that of a gamma-ray photon of the same energy. A beta source placed in a high atomic number metallic shield can produce copious amounts of bremsstrahlung. This is why beta sources are shielded by plastic.

Radioactive materials cannot be turned off. Short half-life radionuclides are often stored in an appropriately shielded location until they have decayed to background. Long-lived radioactive devices (e.g. half-life > 30 days) that have ended their clinical utility are usually disposed of by transfer to an authorized party. The disposal service either recycles the radioactive materials or, more commonly, places them in long-term storage.

Operational and regulatory considerations

Because the potential hazard is higher for therapy than that associated with diagnostic procedures, the corresponding degree of regulatory oversight is more intense. Most jurisdictions require a specific radionuclide license for each type of therapeutic procedure.

Secure control of the radioactive inventory is of special concern. HDR beta or gamma sources are capable of inflicting severe injury from a brief contact. The potential danger of a misplaced device cannot be overstated.

The Nuclear Regulatory Commission (NRC) requires that a qualified physicist (individual with ABR or ABMP certification in therapeutic medical physics) attend all HDR procedures. Medical and technical emergencies will occur from time to time. When this happens, the normal tendency of the medical staff is to focus on the patient. The physicist's responsibility is to remain focused on safely retrieving the sources and minimizing unnecessary exposure of patients and staff.

Radiation instrumentation

Personnel monitoring

Personnel monitoring in a mixed gamma–fluoroscopy field poses new operational and regulatory challenges. Assuming that the effective dose equivalent is the numerical reading of the collar badge makes no allowance for the usual lead apron. Applying a fluoroscopic weighting factor improperly accounts for penetrating gamma-radiation.

Radiation instruments

Two basic radiation instruments are the Geiger-Muller (GM) counter and the ionization chamber survey meter (Figure 26.1). The short response time and audio output of the GM counter provides a rapid indication of source position. The wide sensitivity range of the ion chamber permits accurate measurements under a variety of conditions. Both instruments have their place in the EVBT environment.

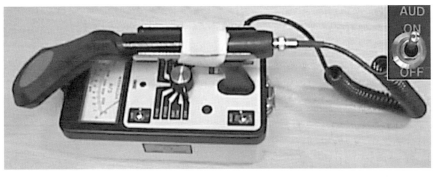

a

Figure 26.1 Examples of a GM counter (a) and an ion-chamber survey meter (b). Note the audio output from the GM instrument.

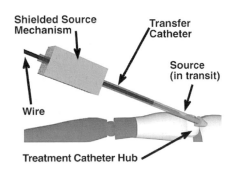

b

219

The GM counter shown in Figure 26.1 is equipped with a beta-sensitive probe. With the ion chamber's plastic beta shield in place, this instrument can only detect gamma-rays and bremsstrahlung. Removing the shield provides beta sensitivity.

Normal treatment—patient safety considerations

The technical objective of a routine removable source treatment is to deliver the source to its assigned location, hold it in position for the prescribed time, and retrieve it into the shielded delivery device. The source irradiates tissue along its insertion and retrieval path. A rapid deployment lowers this transit dose. In general, a slower deployment has a lower probability of mechanical complication.

The principal risk to the patient is the failure to smoothly deploy and retrieve the source. The path in the patient should be routinely tested by deploying and retrieving a dummy source before the actual treatment. An additional benefit of a deployed dummy is the ability to see the 'source' in its treatment position before initiating therapy. The use of dummy sources for removable implants is virtually universal in the practice of cancer brachytherapy.

A 'cool' source increases overall procedure time and might produce an increased frequency of medical complications. A 'warm' source increases the transit dose. It also decreases the time available to detect and correct an abnormality. A 10-min treatment time may be optimum.

Post-treatment considerations

Removing an HDR source from the patient at the end of treatment removes all of the administered radioactive material. The patient is not a radiation hazard. There is no danger for the patient's family or for CCU staff.

Radioactive stents are active until physical decay runs its course. The kBq (μCi) of radioactive materials in stents are not an external radiation hazard.

HDR or LDR patients are occasionally shunned by staff or family because of unwarranted fear of radiation exposure. Staff training together with patient and family counseling mitigates this inappropriate behavior.

Normal treatment—staff safety considerations

Two hypothetical delivery systems are considered for the purposes of this section. These are linear sources of a beta emitter (^{90}Sr/^{90}Y) or a gamma emitter (^{192}Ir). These sources are mounted at the end of a deployment wire

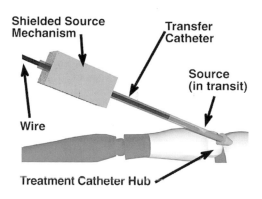

Shielded Source Mechanism

Transfer Catheter

Source (in transit)

Wire

Treatment Catheter Hub

Figure 26.2 The source is stored in a shielded pig. Solid connections to the catheter and an unimpeded delivery path are important.

(Figure 26.2). Either source is brought into the laboratory in a delivery device (pig) that is then connected to the brachytherapy treatment catheter. It is assumed that the device is operated by an individual standing near the pig.

The pig is a source of radiation while the treatment sources are inside. A fraction of the gamma photons leak through the pig's shielding. The leakage intensity is minimized by increasing the thickness of the shielding. Plastic shielding eliminates beta leakage. However, some of the beta particles create bremsstrahlung. In both cases, the operator's hand dose is minimized by not touching the pig.

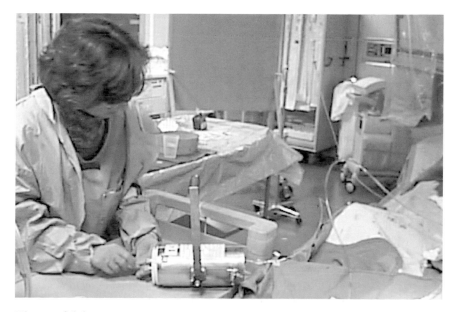

Figure 26.3 The oncologist's position behind the pig reduces her dose.

221

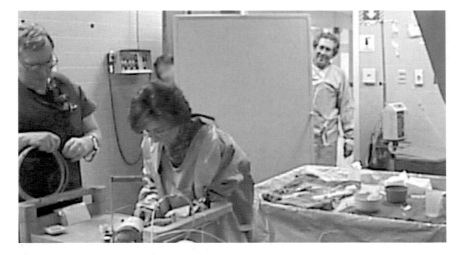

Figure 26.4 *Source loading in progress. The cardiologist is immediately available in case of necessity. Distance and shielding minimize his dose during this process. The door shield is in its typical position.*

The source is deployed from the pig into the patient through the treatment catheter. The source is unshielded for a few seconds during deployment and retrieval. It is important to keep the operator's hands and body away from the treatment catheter during source transit (Figure 26.3). The fluoroscopic apron provides little protection from iridium gamma-rays. There is the possibility that operator dose increases because of beta particle-induced bremsstrahlung in the lead of the fluoroscopic apron. It is useful to employ an appropriate radiation detector with an audible output during source deployment and retrieval. Aural feedback provides a useful safety check on the process.

When the procedure is complete, the patient, laboratory, angiographic equipment, linens, and waste must be surveyed to prevent the loss of a source.

The principles of radiation protection are combined to reduce staff dose to a fraction of the MPD. In the case of individuals outside the laboratory, the objective is maintenance of doses significantly below the public's MPD. (This level corresponds to the difference in natural background between New York and Denver.) In the case of individuals working in the laboratory, the objective is to have a very small fraction of the occupational MPD attributable to brachytherapy.

Once the source is inside the patient, radiation safety issues differ for beta and gamma radionuclides. The patient's tissues fully absorb the beta particles. The only external radiation is bremsstrahlung (produced by interaction of the beta particles with tissue). Iridium gamma photons are typically attenuated by

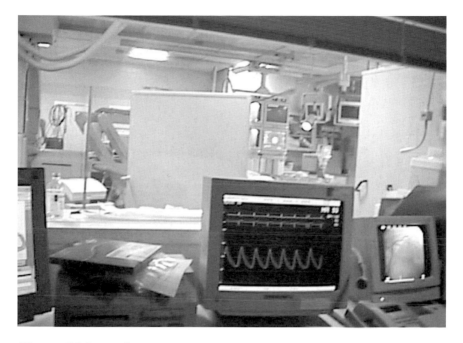

Figure 26.5 *View from the monitoring nurse's position. The shield shadows this space from the radioactive materials in the patient's chest. A video system permits the nurse to observe the patient.*

a factor of two or three. There is a measurable radiation field in the catheterization laboratory and in its environments. What is the practical significance of this radiation field?

We have investigated the situation for iridium HDR treatments. In round numbers, it was determined that the dose delivered to the physicist, oncologist, and cardiologist was < 10 μSv (1 millirem) per procedure. During this experiment, the cardiologist elected to enter the room in approximately half the procedures for reasons such as source position adjustment or assisting the oncologist with the contrast injection manifold. A dose level of 10 μSv is comparable to that received by an interventionist performing a conventional vascular reconstruction.

The dose delivered to an individual standing at the door to our laboratory or sitting in the control room is < 5 μSv per procedure (Figure 26.4). Auxiliary therapy shields (25 mm of lead) reduce this to < 0.5 μSv per procedure (Figure 26.5). Given these values, an unshielded individual could stand at the door for > 200 procedures per year without exceeding the general public's MPD. Remaining behind the auxiliary shield increases this to > 2000 procedures per year.

Emergency conditions—patient safety considerations

A medical event is the most likely emergency event. The source should be immediately returned to the pig when this occurs. This should be done by the authorized user. The physicist should be appropriately trained and prepared to retrieve the source if necessary.

Prolonged deployment or retrieval is an expected technical emergency. This can produce an unwanted dose to tissues along the catheter track and might produce an excessive staff dose. The physicist should monitor deployment time and advise immediate removal if deployment is prolonged. Prolonged retrieval may be more difficult. The first backup procedure is to withdraw the entire treatment catheter from the patient and place the source plus catheter into an appropriate bail-out box (Figure 26.6). Depending upon the catheter location and the experience of the authorized user, this may have to be done by the catheterizing physician.

Failure to retrieve the source from the patient is an extremely low probability event with serious potential consequences. The physicist's survey of the patient and equipment after treatment is the first line of defense against leaving a source in the patient. The immediate action should be an attempt to move the source into a larger diameter artery. Surgical backup should be

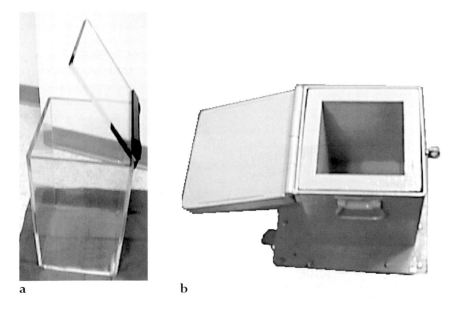

a   b

Figure 26.6 *Plastic beta (a) and lead gamma (b) bail-out boxes. These large containers provide a location for emergency source disposal. The appropriate box must be in the laboratory during every procedure.*

224

called while the angiographer attempts source retrieval using standard percutaneous instruments. Emergency surgery is the final level of backup for this emergency.

Switching to fluid sources: balloons might leak or burst and spill their contents into the patient's bloodstream. The radioactive materials need to be physiologically cleared from the patient before an unacceptable dose is delivered to any tissue. A gaseous ^{133}Xe spill is rapidly exhaled and presents minimum radiation hazard to the patient. The chemical form of radioactive liquids is chosen for rapid excretion in case of a spill. Should this occur, the critical organ dose (bowel or bladder) is acceptable.

Any technical malfunction, even one involving a dummy source, should be reported to the manufacturer and, if required, to the regulatory authorities. The resulting database serves to detect patterns of malfunction. This might prevent disastrous consequences.

Emergency conditions—staff safety considerations

If the source is retrieved promptly, there should be no additional staff dose attributable to a medical emergency. Preplanning and rehearsal are essential to meet this goal.

Solid sources
Direct finger contact with an HDR source is extremely hazardous. By their very nature, such sources are capable of producing major skin burns in a few moments. The emergency kit (Figure 26.7), which is required to be in the

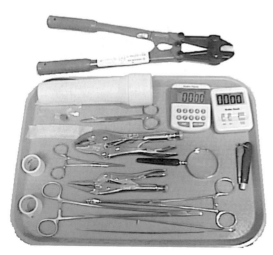

Figure 26.7 *Operational and emergency tray for a wire-based HDR system. An assortment of long-handled instruments minimizes the need to touch a source. The tools can be used to manipulate stuck parts of the delivery device. The bolt cutter is available to deal with a snarled wire. The flashlight permits operation should the lights fail. Redundant timers minimize certain treatment errors.*

room during each procedure, must contain appropriate instruments for grasping a source. The smallest such instruments should provide a spacing of at least 10 cm between the source and the user's hand. Longer distances are desirable.

Staff dose resulting from events that end up with the source and its delivery device being promptly placed in the bail-out box should be low. This assumes that the team keeps their hands and bodies well away from the known or estimated source position. Long instruments are particularly valuable in this regard.

Staff dose resulting from the retrieval of stuck or lost sources will be higher. Even when such an unlikely event occurs, it is unlikely that the MPD will be exceeded. Here again, long instruments protect the operator's hands. If such an event occurs, the hand and body radiation monitors of all team members should be sent out for immediate reading. It is prudent, therefore, for the entire team to always wear their dosimeters.

Gaseous and liquid sources

A laboratory performing ^{133}Xe procedures needs to have adequate ventilation to rapidly exhaust the contaminated air outside the hospital. The design also needs to provide sufficient dilution to protect those individuals living or working near the exhaust.

A spilled liquid source can radioactively contaminate the laboratory along with the clothing and skin of staff members. The laboratory may have to be closed for days if the contamination cannot be removed. It is conceivable that a staff member might ingest some of the liquid and become internally contaminated. The excreta of a contaminated patient can produce further contamination. There are standard radiation safety procedures for dealing with radioactive contamination.

Concluding remarks

The choice of an optimum radiation source and its delivery technology is still a matter of research. Some safety measures are specific to a particular system. Others are of more general applicability. A knowledgable team is essential to minimize risk.

FURTHER READING

Allen J, Taylor, Patrick D et al. Long-term coronary vascular response to^{32}P β-particle-emitting stents in a canine model. *Circulation* 1999; **100**:2366–2372.

Amols HI, Trichter F, Weinberger J. Intracoronary radiation for prevention of restenosis: dose perturbations caused by stents. *Circulation* 1998; **98**:2024–2029.

Apple MG. XenaCath dosimetry and radio safety profile. Data and results on File: 1996. Cook Inc. Personal communication.

Atkins HL, Robertson JF, Croft BY et al. Estimates of radiation absorbed doses from radioxenons in lung imaging. *J Nuclear Med* 1980; **21**:459.

Balter S. Endovascular brachytherapy: physics and technology. *Cathet Cardiovasc Diagn* 1998; **45**:292–298.

Bhargava B, Vodovotz Y, Waksman R. Intracoronary radiation therapy for prevention of restenosis. *Indian Heart J* 1998, **50**(Suppl):120 129.

Calfee RV, Ali N, Bradshaw T, Raizner A. The NeoCardia system for restenosis prevention. In: Waksman R, King SB, Crocker IR, Mould RF, eds. *Vascular Brachytherapy*. AX Veenendaal, Nucletron BV: The Netherlands, 1996:338–342.

Carlier SG, Marijinissen JP, Coen VL, et al. Guidance of intracoronary radiation therapy based on dose-volume histograms derived from quantitative intravascular ultrasound. *IEEE Trans Med Imaging* 1998; **17**:772–778.

Carter AJ, Scott D, Bailey L, Hoopes T, Jones R, Virmani R. Dose-response effects of ^{32}P radioative stents in an atherosclerotic porcine coronary model. *Circulation* 1999; **100**:1548–1531.

Carter JC, Laird RJ, Bailey LR et al. Effects of endovascular radiation from a β particle-emitting stent in a porcine coronary restenosis model: a dose–response study. *Circulation* 1996; **94**:2364–2368.

Chiu-Tsao ST, de la Zerda A, Lin J et al. High sensitivity gatchromic film dosimetry for I-125 seed. *Med Phys* 1994; **21**:651–657.

Choppin G, Rydberg J, Lilhjenzin JO. *Radiochemistry and Nuclear Chemistry*, 2nd edn. Butterworth-Heinemann: Oxford, 1995.

Costa MA, Sabat M, van der Giessen WJ et al. Late coronary occlusion after intracoronary brachytherapy. *Circulation* 1999; **100**:789–792.

Diamond DA, Vesely TM. The role of radiation therapy in the management of vascular restenosis. Part II. Radiation techniques and results. *J Vasc Interv Radiol* 1998; **9**:389–400.

Diamond DA, Vesely TM. Therapy in the management of vascular restenosis. Part II. Radiation techniques and results. *J Vasc Interv Radiol* 1998; **9**:389–400.

Dupont/Merck, Radiopharmaceutical Division. Package Insert Label: Xenon-133 Gas, March 1994.

Evans RD. *The Atomic Nucleus.* McGraw Hill: New York, 1955.

Fischell TA. Radioactive stents. *Semi Interv Cardiol* 1998; **3**:51–56.

Fischell TA, Hehrlein C. The radioisotope stent for the prevention of restenosis. *Herz* 1998; **23**:373–379.

Greiner RH, Do DD, Mahler F et al. Peripheral endovascular radiation for restenosis after percutaneous transluminal angioplasty (PTA). *1998 Endovascular Brachytherapy Workshop.* Napoli, Italy, May 10, 1998.

Hehrlein C, Kaiser S, Riessen R, Metz J, Fritz P, Kubler W. External beam radiation after stent implantation increases neointimal hyperplasia by augmenting smooth muscle cell proliferation and extracellularl matrix accumulation. *J Am Coll Cardiol* 1999; **34**:561–566.

International Commission on Radiation Units and Measurements. *Radiation Quantities and Units*, Report 33. ICRU/NCRP Publications: Bethesda, 1980.

Jani SK. Data on brachytherapy dosimetry. In: *Handbook of Dosimetry Data for Radiotherapy.* CRC Press: Boca Raton, FL, 1993:150–151.

Jani SK. Basic physics of gamma isotopes. In: Waksman R, ed. *Vascular Brachytherapy*, 2nd edn. Futura Publishing: Armonk, NY, 1999:167–176.

Jani SK. Physics of vascular brachytherapy. *J Inv Cardiol* 1999; **11**.

Jani SK, Massullo VM, Teirstein PS et al. Physics and safety aspects of a coronary irradiation pilot study to inhibit restenosis using manually loaded Ir-192 ribbons. *Semin Intervent Cardiol* 1997; **2**:119–124.

Kaluza GL, Ali NM, Abukhalil JM, Waksman R, Oesterle SN, Raizner AE. Intracoronary beta-radiation is equally effective after stenting and balloon angioplasty: a subanalysis of the PREVENT trial. *Am J Cardiol* 1999 (in press).

King SB, Williams DO, Chougule P et al. Endovascular beta-radiation to reduce restenosis after coronary balloon angioplasty: results of the beta energy restenosis trial. *Circulation* 1998; **97**:2025–2030.

Knoll GF. *Radiation Detection and Measurement*, 2nd edn. Wiley & Sons: New York, 1989.

Lansky AJ, Popma JJ, Massullo V et al. Radiation to inhibit intimal proliferation post stenting (SCRIPPS) trial. *Am J Cardiol* 1999; **84**:410–414.

228

Lavie E, Kijel D, Sayag E *et al*. Pre-clinical experience with a radioactive rhenium (Re186/Re188) catheter based-system. *3rd International Meeting on Interventional Cardiology*, Jerusalem, 1999:37 (abstract).

Leo WR. *Techniques for Nuclear and Particle Physics Experiments*. Springer-Verlag: Berlin, 1992.

Liermann D, Kirchner J, Bauernsachs R, Schopohl B, Bottcher HD. Brachytherapy with iridium-912 HDR to prevent from restenosis in peripheral *Herz* 1995; **76**:112–116.

Liermann D, Bauernsachs R, Schopohl B, Bottcher HD. Five year follow-up after brachytherpy for restenosis in peripheral arteries. *Semi Interv Cardiol* 1997; **2**:133–137.

Limpijankit T, Waksman R, Yock PG, Fitzgerald PJ. Intravascular ultrasound volumetric assessment of intimal hyperplasia in stents treated with intracoronary radiation. *Am J Cardiol* 1999; **84**:850–858.

Mazur W, Ali NM, Debaghi SF et al. High dose rate intracoronary radiation suppresses neointimal proliferation in the stented and ballooned model of porcine restenosis. *Circulation* 1994;**90**:I-652.

Mazur W, Ali NM, Khan MM et al. High dose rate intracoronary radiation for inhibition of neointimal formation in the stented and balloon-injured porcine models of restenosis: angiographic, morphometric and histopathologic analyses. *Int J Radiat Oncol Biol Phys* 1996; **36**:777–778.

Meerkin D, Radif JC, Crocker IR et al. Effects of intracoronary beta-radiation therapy after coronary angioplasty: an intravscular ultrasound study. *Circulation* 1999; **99**:1660–1665.

Minar E, Pokrajac B, Ahmadi R, et al. Brachytherpy for prophylaxis of restenosis after long-segment femoropopliteal angioplasty: pilot study. *Radiology* 1998; **208**:173–179.

National Council on Radiation Protection and Measurements. In: Mann WB, ed. *A Handbook of Radioactivity Measurements Procedures*, Report No. 58, 2nd edn. NCRP Publications: Bethesda, 1985.

Nori D, Parikh S, Moni J. Management of peripheral vascular disease: innovative approaches using radiation therapy. *Int J Radiat Oncol Biol Phys* 1996; **36**:847–856.

Parikh S, Nori D. Endovascular brachytherapy: current status and future trends. *J Brachyther Int* 1997; **13**:167–177.

Pokrajac B, Minar E, Knocke TH et al. HDR-brachytherapy for prophylaxis of restenosis after femoropopliteal angioplasty: results from a randomized trial—Vienna 02. *1998 Endovascular Brachytherapy Workshop*. Napoli, Italy, May 10, 1998.

Popowski Y, Verin V, Papirov I et al. High dose rate brachytherapy for prevention of restenosis after percutaneous transluminal coronary angioplasty. Preliminary dosimetric tests of a new source presentation. *Int J Radiat Oncol Biol Phys* 1995;**33**:211–215.

229

Popowski Y, Verin V, Papirov I et al. Intra-arterial 90-yttrium brachytherapy. Preliminary dosimetric study using a specially modified angioplasty balloon. *Int J Radiat Oncol Biol Phys* 1995;**33**:713–717.

Popowski Y, Verin V, Schwager M et al. A novel system for intracoronary β-irradiation: description and dosimetric results. *Int J Radiat Oncol Biol Phys* 1996;**36**:923–931.

Popowski Y, Verin V, Urban P et al. Intra-arterial yttrium-90 brachytherapy for restenosis prevention. In: Mould GB, Mould RF, eds. *Freiburg Oncology Series, Brachytherapy Review*, Monograph no. 1. Albert-Ludwigs-University: Freiburg, Germany, 1994:163–165.

Popowski Y, Verin V, Urban P. Endovascular β-irradiation after percutaneous transluminal coronary balloon angioplasty. *Int J Radiat Oncol Biol Phys* 1996;**36**:841–845.

Raizner AE, Ali NM, Kaluza GL, Abukhalil JM. Therapeutic window of intracoronary beta-radiation dose with 32P in humans: dose range analysis from the PREVENT trial. *Circulation* 1999 (in press).

Raizner AE, Calfee RV. The Guidant intravascular brachytherapy system. In: Waksman R, Serruys PW, eds. *Handbook of Vascular Brachytherapy*. Martin Dunitz: London, 1998.

Raizner AE, Calfee RV, Ali MN, Bradshaw AJ, Eno RP. The Guidant coronary source wire system. In: *Vascular Brachytherapy*, 2nd edn. Futura Publishing: Armonk, NY, 1999:505–519.

Raizner AE, Mazur W, Ali MN et al. Endovascular gamma radiation using HDR in the swine model. In: Waksman R, King SB, Crocker IR, Mould RF, eds. *Vascular Brachytherapy*. Nucletron BV: AX Veenendaal, The Netherlands, 1996:154–164.

Raizner AE, Oesterle S, Waksman R et al. The PREVENT trial: a feasibility study of intracoronary brachytherapy in the prevention of restenosis: an interim report. *Circulation* 1998; **98**:I-651.

Raizner AE, Oesterle S, Waksman R et al. Inhibition of restenosis with beta-emitting radiation (^{32}P): the final report of the PREVENT trial. *Circulation* 1999 (in press).

Reynaert N, Verhaegen F, Taeymans Y, van Eijkeren M, Thierens H. Monte Carlo calculations of dose distributions around ^{32}P and ^{198}Au stents for intravascular brachytherapy. *Med Phys* 1999; **26**:1484–1491.

Sabate M, Kay IP, van Der Giessen WJ et al. Preserved endothelium-dependent vasodilation in coronary segments previously treated with balloon angioplasty and intracoronary irradiation. *Circulation* 1999; **100**:1623–1629.

Sabate M, Serruys PW, van Der Giessen WJ et al. Geometric vascular remodeling after balloon angioplasty and beta-radiation therapy: A three-dimensional intravascular ultrasound study. *Circulation* 1999; **100**:1182–1188.

Schopohl B, Liermann D, Pohlit LJ et al. Ir-192 endovascular brachytherapy for avoidance of intimal hyperplasia after percutaneous transluminal angioplasty and stent implantation in peripheral vessels: 6 years experience. *Int J Radiat Oncol Biol Phys* 1996; **36**:835–840.

Umm AR, Mon EH, Koytor F. *Und talat ditum*. Martin Dunitz: London, 2000.

Shiran A, Mintz GS, Waksman R et al. Early lumen loss after treatment of in-stent restenosis: an intravascular ultrasound study. *Circulation* 1998; **98**:200–203.

Teirstein PS. Beta radiation to reduce restenosis – too little, too soon? *Circulation* 1997; **95**:1095–1097.

Teirstein PS, Massullo VM, Jani SK et al. Catheter-based radiotherapy to inhibit restenosis after coronary stenting. *N Engl J Med* 1997; **336**:1697–1703.

Teirstein S, Massullo V, Jani S et al. Two-year follow-up after catheter-based radiotherapy to inhibit coronary restenosis. *Circulation* 1996; **99**:243–247.

Teirstein PS. Vascular radiation therapy: the devil is in the dose. *J Am Coll Cardiol* 1999; **34**:567–569.

Trerotola SO, Carmody TJ, Timmerman RD et al. Brachytherapy for the preventon of stenosis in a canine hemodialysis graft model: preliminary observations. *Radiology* 1999; **212**:748–54.

Tripuraneni P, Giap H, Jani S. Endovascular brachytherapy for peripheral vascular disease. *Semin Rad Oncol* 1999; **9**:190–202.

Verin V, Popowski Y, Urban P et al. Intraarterial beta irradiation prevents neointimal hyperplasia in a hypercholesterolemic rabbit restenosis model. *Circulation* 1995;**92**:2284–2290.

Verin V, Urban P, Popowski Y et al. Feasibility of intracoronary beta irradiation to reduce restenosis after balloon angioplasty. A clinical pilot study. *Circulation* 1997;**95**:1138–1144.

Waksman R. Endovascular radiation therapy for the peripheral vascular system. In: Waksman R, King SB, Crocker IR, Mould RF, eds. *Vascular Brachytherapy*. The Nucletron BV: Netherlands, 1996:273–278.

Waksman R. Current status of vascular radiotherapy: U.S. pilot studies. *Proceedings of the International Seminar on the Current Status of Radiotherapy in the World: Brachytherapy in the Next Millennium*, New York, April 17–19, 1997.

Waksman R. Endovascular brachytherapy: overcoming 'practical' obstacles. *Am J Cardiol* 1998; **81**:21E–26E.

Waksman R. Intracoronary brachytherapy: overcoming 'practical' obstacles. *Herz* 1998; **23**:401–406.

Waksman R, Chan RC, Vodovotz Y, Bass BG, Apple MG. Radioactive 133-Xenon gas-filled angioplasty balloon: A novel intracoronary radiation system to prevent restenosis. *J Am Coll Cardiol* 1998; **31**:2 356A.

Waksman R. Late thrombosis after radiation, Sitting on a time bomb. *Circulation* 1999; **100**:780–782.

Wardeh AJ, Kay IP, Sabate M et al. Beta-particle-emitting radioactive stent implantation. A safety and feasibility study. *Circulation* 1999; **100**:1684–1689.

Weinberger J. Intracoronary radiation using radioisotope solution-filled balloons. *Herz* 1998; **23**:366–372.

Wilcox J, Waxman R, King SB et al. The role of the adventitia in the arterial response to angioplasty: the effect of intravascular radiation. *Int J Radiat Oncol Biol Phys* **36**:789–796.

INDEX